Blonde **Blues:**
Sex, Intimacy, More Sex, and One More Thing!

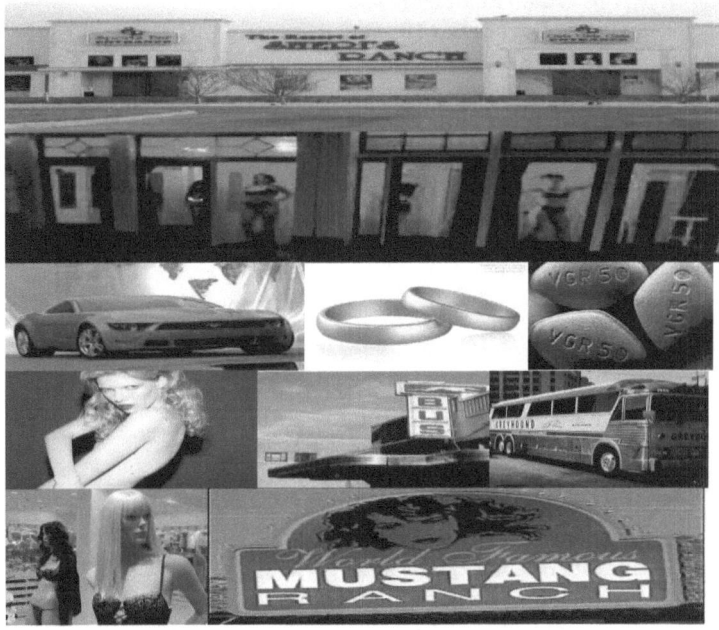

AN ADULT ROMANCE
NOVEL

Bryce Condon
USA & EU Copyright 2010 - 2020

INTRODUCTION

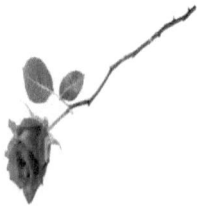

INTRODUCTION:

Suppose you had only a few months left in your dull and sexually deprived life; a life that you always went by the book, and with most strict interpretation of it; a life with a lot of inhibitions that were self imposed or were drilled into your brain. You lived, but you never dared to have fun. Every time an attractive woman caught your attention, your inflamed passion was aroused. However, you had incarcerated yourself into "Look, but do not touch" Victorian jail.

However, now that you have only a short time to live, you decide to really live it up and cram in a lot of those passionate, sex life pleasures and fulfillments that you never had! Think that you decide to live all those fantasies, pleasures, and the good life that you or others denied you. Imagine being free of everyday life pressures and stresses. Then imagine that you give yourself permission and blessing to live that perfect sex, passion, and intimate life like you see on Hollywood movie screens.

Think that if your life was a Hollywood movie, you can now in these last few months remaining in your life rewrite it so you will not be caught on your deathbed dreadfully thinking "What if I did in fact do what I dreamed and fanaticized to do all my dull life? What if I had permitted myself to live?"

This book shows you how you could do all of these pleasures legally and as gentleman and to your heart's content? I did them in my real life, you can too, and now I tell you all about it.

This book lifts you up like a rocket and puts you right in the middle of romantic and sexual fantasies that you did not even permit yourself to dream. These are dreams of having that perfect sex with the most beautiful women in the world and under the most perfect conditions with no worries and no negative consequences.

This is the feelings that the Hollywood movie stars pretend on the screen to feel and touch, but you will feel and sense them in your imagination in vivid color and as if in actual life reality.

Then there is the question of "And then what?" This is where in your rewritten movie, you go back to your real life, back to your real self and surroundings after all that sex, excitement, romance, and pleasure. This is where a more satisfied you starts to re-enter your life as it actually is, right here and right now! Believe me; you will not look at your life the same way after you have read this book. This is because this book frees you from those pent-up feelings of not having had a great, passionate, and intimate sex life.

The answer to "And then what?" is given as "And one more thing" adding to your complete fulfillment in later chapters!

Sex, Intimacy, More Sex, and One More Thing!

I had just listened to my internist's telephone message. His message put fear of God in my heart. Before listening to all of it, I felt an intense rage that was complicated by disgust and a feeling of eternal hopelessness.

I did have a well educated and outstanding cardiologist. However, his antagonist who was my internist had both tried to warn me before. Regrettably, this time they meant serious and life threatening business. My heart attack of a few years ago had now sentenced me to have diagnostic angiogram as well as severe running stress test.

My chiropractor had also threatened me about the serious lower back problem. He had ordered me to lose about twenty to thirty pounds. My extra weight had undone some of his careful treatment, and had "rendered it utterly useless." He was upset and disappointed that I had, intentionally or unintentionally gained some weight rather than losing. My lower back pain had made every movement painful. To carry on daily motions of walking and sitting, I had to take heavy doses of painkillers.

The blood pressure pills prescribed by the cardiologist had pretty much "rendered" me impotent. However, the internist had prescribed Viagra but cautioned me that I should not take the Nitroglycerin tablets with Viagra. Nitroglycerin tablets can save lives in the event of heart attack if they are taken under the tongue. However, if I take Viagra to be good enough to function in bed, just to function, the combination of Viagra and Nitroglycerin could kill me.

"Being good enough in bed?" Crying out loud, this meant that sex equals death! What a contrast to when I had sex one, two, or even three times a day. This was a death sentence to a man who spent two weeks in the Red Light District of Amsterdam having sex with most beautiful blondes, brunettes, and shiny black haired ladies one after another.

If I was sentenced to be confined to a wheelchair soon, or die, then I wanted to have my "Last Tango in Paris". Marlon Brando won several academy awards for this film. However, I had never seen the movie or the book. Nevertheless the title was luring enough to imagine one last pleasurable fun. I longed for one last splurge, one last fling, and one last orgasm before I could not any more. The honest truth is that the title had wrongly captured my imagination. I had always liked Marlon Brando. He is an outstanding actor. However, it was only after the first edition of this book that I really and carefully watched the entire movie.

I must say that I was appalled with this movie. In spite the super acting, cinematography, music, and everything, I could not stomach the forced and violent sex acts shown in this movie.

However, to its credit, this movie powerfully depicts what a sexual addict is. This movie shows what perverts and rapists feel and do. This book is about gentle, caring, yet intensely fun sex between two consenting adults as opposed to rape which is a criminal act.

Another movie that is interesting is "Lie with me". The story is about a young and beautiful All American girl from somewhere in the Midwest. I bought this DVD because of its sexy cover. The cover design is similar to the "Last Tango in Paris"; it has the same sexy coloration and style. There are many sex acts in this movie and one real gut ranching scene. This awful scene is about when the mother has to tell her the teenage girl that she has decided to leave her father since there is no sex and no intimacy in their marriage any more. This breaks the heart of the girl. This is so painful for her that when she gets older, she does not seem to enjoy sex. As a result sex, intimacy, and relationships are painful emotionally for her. Hollywood somehow portrays sex as some dangerous and strange thing. I have yet to find a decent movie about a man and woman making love and enjoying it. Most of the sex seems to border around rape, assault, dysfunction, and perversion.

Some research indicates that most American prostitutes are either victims of incest, rape, mutilation, or are from broken families. In Europe, and especially Holland, this is not the case. Legalized prostitution did have some positive things for Holland.

In one of the later chapters, my son gets into a quagmire of divorce. Just like the "Lie with Me", his children end up suffering all their lives.

As these thoughts were going through my mind, I started to go back to the fact that I had only a few quarters to live and I wanted to have gentle, as loving as possible sex. I wanted it to be legal so I went to Holland and Sheri's Ranch in Pahrump, Nevada near Las Vegas. Incidentally, prostitution is not legal in Las Vegas! However, most importantly, I had zero tolerance for any S&M or sexual dysfunctional or violence.

Nevertheless, since I was to live a short time, even AIDS had become a small worry since I knew that it took time for AIDS to kill. I was going to die anyway. So, it really did not matter.

AIDS, which had frightened me before, could not scare me anymore! AIDS had been one major reason for my not trying even the simplest of sexual gratification with other women than my wife before. Of course, protected sex is safe, or as safe as it can be. However, all those years I had been scared to death of visiting sex workers because of AIDS. Now, if I was supposed to die, then the matter was mute. Although horrified before, thoughts of one last splurge helped me to be no longer scared. Now I was free from this awfully terrifying disease since, I would be dying anyways.

I was fifty nine years old that month, and married to a mostly frigid and menopausal wife whom I nevertheless loved, and loved dearly. It seemed like our marriage started as a belligerent argument in our honeymoon that persisted for the twenty-two lingering and dull years of our entire marriage; Married for good, since we had two children together; Married for the bad, since there was almost never any intimacy or sexual gratification for either side; Until death do us apart! When my wife reached fifty, she started to notice the same facial wrinkles in her face that I had noticed for many years. By nature, she is secretive and not talkative. In the same vein, it seemed like she wanted to keep these obvious wrinkles a secret too. Paradoxically, these same wrinkles had made my pure love for her even more everlasting. Surprisingly, at the same time, these wrinkles were a source of relief to her since fifty meant no more matrimonial obligation for the curse of sex; even though there had never been much of passionate sex or intimacy before.

As my old beat up car screeched to a grudging stop near our house, I was one hot defiant, outraged, and remorseful dirty old man. Luckily, Grace Slick's song from Jefferson Airplane was blasting in my head so loud that it drenched all the feelings of defeat and deficiency. The song says, "Do not let them catch you facing down!"

Hell no, I won't be caught face down, no matter how old, or how sick I was!

Years of therapy with several therapists had not resolved my "sex puzzle" dilemma. That was until, finally I found my present therapist. She is a tall and gorgeous European natural blonde with light turquoise blue eyes. She reads a lot of books, and is extremely effective. She is strikingly attractive. Attractive enough to be a movie star with all the glamour associated with it. Many times her soothing, yet insightful, powerful words had comforted me in some of the most difficult stages of my life. Her stunning beauty, warmth, intelligence, had melted away my life's deep sadness.

In my grief, loneliness, and depression, being alone in the same room with my therapist who is one of the sexiest, intelligent, and desirable women in the world convinced me that I needed her. I needed her warm and understanding companion and therapy in the isolation that I was feeling; I needed her professional care that helped me cope. Especially now, I needed her supportive analysis that had made a big difference many times before. I urgently needed this because I knew I was going to do some daring wild living in the last few months of my life just like I had done when I was young. I badly needed her as a safety net, as a voice of sanity in a fatally insane situation.

Emphatically enough, she remains a professional who is totally distant and who would not even touch my hand for a handshake. I have fantasized about her numerous times. My fantasies were not just for sex. My fantasies were about us being happily married together. Something that will never happen in million years let alone in a few remaining months of my painful life.

As usual, the dinner at home was one of the self-serve types. Plenty of frozen TV dinners in the freezer, along with leftovers in the refrigerator, were pleading for me to warm them up for dinner. My wife and kids had already heated up their rock solid, aluminum packaged dinners an hour before. They even had the courtesy to clean the table.

I watched the evening news with my wife and then went to bed without exchanging a word. However, before making it to my bed, she repeated her damning phrase that "We are just like a roommate; you cannot call this a marriage; you are loser; you will never know what to do with a woman." She had no idea about my death sentence and I was damned if I told her. I was dying and my wife and I had never had anything resembling warmth or emotional closeness of a normal marriage.

Just to drive the message home, she added that she will soon get a divorce attorney …

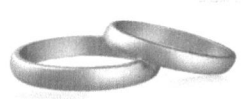 CHAPTER 2: My First Loves

Prior to that suffocating telephone message from my cardiologist, I had had an incredibly lucky, exciting, and daring life. As a single man I cherished women. Each woman was worthy of love, affection, and potential for being a nurturing mother, girlfriend, just plain friend, wife, companion, or even just to watch. I had even made a major discovery in the third grade.

In the third grade, I was sitting right next to a pretty girl exactly my age. Since this was a bench seat, and I was the middle student on it, my right thy sometimes would inadvertently touch the pretty girl's left thy. However, when the same touching happened with the boy on the other side, I did my best to quickly correct that situation and pull myself closer to the girl. This touch sensation felt good with girl, but it felt eerily with the boy.

Our teacher was from a well known family and she always dressed well. She always had an elegant hair style. I was her most favorite student since I always did my homework and was great in Math. She had lived in Europe several years. Furthermore, her sister was a flight attendant for SAS in Sweden. One day she showed us her sister's picture. She was even prettier than our teacher.

My first love was a half Persian and Half French girl named Roya. In Persian Roya means dream. The summer that we met, her parents were vacationing in South of France and she had to stay with her French grandmother to finish her last test and then join them after three weeks. She was seventeen and I was twenty one.

Her grandmother was best friends with my mother. My mother had always adored Roya and had told her grandmother about this several times. So one day all four of us went to a Café to have tea and coffee. One look and I was in love. Her grandmother, being a French Resistance fighter of World War II, and a Widow who lost her husband in the war, also knew that I was a good man. I had just graduated with Honors, and I looked very presentable with a tailor-made suite. In addition, I weighed the perfect weight for my height. My mother arranged for a chaperoned date two days later. The rules, as per her absent parents, and according to French law was that we were allowed to be together under grandmother's, or my mother's supervision at all times.

In perfect compliance with the French Rules of Conduct, we ended up going to the same café several times each week. My mother and her grandmother would sit at one table and we would sit at another.

Roya was very interested about my life story. She had jet black hair adorned with an unpretentious gold tiara. She was passionate but she conducted herself according the code of behavior expected from her absent parents and she was very lady like.

On the second date, we had our first kiss when her grandmother went to open the door. This kiss was nothing like all the other kisses that I had before. This one had sealed my heart for Roya.

She spoke in lyrics, and she was a poet in her own right. Roya's dream was to design fashion dresses under her own label and sell them in her own boutique. She was also quite serious about having three kids.

We proposed and decided to get married in a year or two. We were in love! Every part of my body and soul longed for her. I had collected as many things as I could from my chaperoned dates with her. I had a notebook that was dedicated to our romance and love. There were pictures of her; her poems including one about me; a newspaper article about the right way to parent children; a pamphlet showing our favorite café; a copy of US Army "Dos and Don'ts of Dating"; several swatches of cloth material that she intended to design her dresses with.

We also had planned our life together. She will buy me a Fire Engine Red Ford Mustang when I got to the ripe age of forty. The age forty was considered the age when men went crazy and bought a sports car as a treatment for the mid life crisis. The three weeks went by in a blink of an eye, and we went to the airport to see her off on the Air France flight to Paris. We did get to have a long hug, and a big kiss before her departure. I called her twice each week, even though it was quite expensive those days. Unfortunately, her mother for whatever reason had been dead set against our relationship. She had dismissed it from the beginning by saying we were just too young for such a big commitment as marriage. This had put her mother on one side, and my mother and her grandmother on the other side. "This is true love as it can be" my mother would say. "My son is a good man, ask anyone." And to confirm, her grandmother would add that "Bryce is a gentleman. Let us not lose this chance. I testify that they are love birds, and in addition he is a mature and well behaved twenty-one year-old."

A few weeks later, my father and her father both doctors got together for lunch. This lunch time "Consultation", which is what Doctors routinely do to discuss important things about their patients, was put together to help their kids. Both my parents, and hers, had noticed that we were seriously lovesick!

In addition to realization of love sickness in me, they had felt that they had an obligation towards me. We had an unspoken agreement that if I was a gentleman, got an excellent education, and staid clean, they do their best to help. Help me with getting married with my dream girl. Well Roya meant that dream girl, and almost all of us were convinced that she was my dream girl.

My dad came home somewhat sad after the consultation. His only advice was, "I wanted to marry your mother, and nothing stopped me", then somewhat uncharacteristically he added the French proverb that said something like, "All is fair in war and love!"

I still was excited about Roya's return from vacation in France after two weeks.

When Roya's Air France landed, we were not in the airport. Her grandmother had given two convincing reasons to my mother to prevent us from going. One was that she was very angry with her daughter and son in-law. Two, for Roya's broken heart sake.

Roya did call me as soon as she and her parents had arrived home. She had brought me a shirt and a coffee cup and saucer as a keepsake and reminder of those times we met in the café. We exchanged love letters for a few months, but then, she stopped.

Not getting those love letters made me feel depressed. Nothing could help me get over my intense longing for love, intimacy, and sex with Roya. However, so long as the letters were coming, I had some dim hope. Unfortunately, when the letters stopped, the craving got worse than ever before. How could this happen? In her last letter, she talked about "The Barber of Civil" opera. This is a love story that is destroyed by betrayal of a family member. This opera has an excellent Aria that always reminds me of Roya. It almost always brings tears in my eyes. Roya was four years younger than I.

After all these years, I still wonder how our marriage would have been like.

There is a saying that God has a sense of humor. God's sense of humor is not always happy to us human beings, but nevertheless funny in retrospect. A few years later, fate or God's sense of humor, resulted in my getting a summer job in New York City a block or so away from Fifth Ave. which is the Mecca for pretty women and boutiques. The same Fifth Ave. that Roya dreamed of opening a boutique.

During my lunch hour, I spend a lot of my time looking for "Roya Boutique" that was never there. I know it. However, I hoped that someday I magically see it open. I even managed to get a date with one of those most beautiful women in the world.

I was lovesick. I wanted to make love to Roya. I wanted it to be Roya forever!

Of course, I was young and testosterones were jumping inside. I would have dreams of going to the honeymooner's paradise hotel somewhere in secluded romantic setting in Pennsylvania. I saw her in my dreams with the wedding dress that she had told me she liked.

The sex drive, in addition to depression got too much to handle. Two weeks before going back to college that summer, I decided to take advantage of super low standby tickets offered by TWA. I hopped on a New York to London flight. Once in Heathrow Airport, I noticed that I could fly to Amsterdam with KLM for 65% less than the usual price.

I was on my way to visit one of my best friends from the high school who had married a Dutch woman and was teaching in Utrecht Historical University. A fifty-three year old businessman was sitting next to me. He was on a business trip to Amsterdam. He pointed out the sightseeing places in Amsterdam. He mentioned the Red Light District as where the most beautiful prostitutes (or sex-workers, as he called them) were. He pointed out that it was legal, and it was clean.

Being a man, and somewhat observant from religion point of view, I dismissed the idea. Yet a few days later, I decided to give Red Light District a try as a way of numbing my hurt feelings of pain for losing Roya.

As Sir Richard Branson of the Virgin Atlantic Airline would say it, I lost my virginity. In fact I lost my virginity in the Red Light District. Nevertheless, at the end of those two weeks and lots of sex with sexual artists, I still had a mixture of pains of loss, emptiness, and serenity combined with euphoria. After all, I had been with the most beautiful women in the world. That alone should have been the most satisfying thing, if not the only thing in this world as per Hollywood.

Nevertheless, sex, even saturation sex did not seem to lead to complete euphoria it was visually and enticingly ingrained on the movie screens.

Just like everyone else, I too grew up on watching perfect images of painted ladies and gentlemen in an ideal looking set on TV. Thus, as a child, these images had brainwashed me into sincerely believing that there was some sort of elixir-like heavenly delight in having an orgasm with a perfect blue-eyed blonde, Play Boy centerfold. Nothing else would come close to this ultimate delight.

On the screen, many perfect looking painted gentlemen seemed to risk their lives and do heroics just so at the end they make love to that gorgeous blonde who was equally passionate and loved and equally lusted for those testosterone-fueled gentlemen adventures and they really liked the sex; sex was not dirty; sex was equally exhilarating to men and women.

This childhood brainwashing was so profound that I was experiencing a post traumatic syndrome that was based on the decades of deprivation I felt for not having that ultimate blonde experience. It also clearly seemed to me that everyone else seemed to have that sex and I could not!

However, from a spiritual sense, I did subconsciously know that body, soul, and mind can and usually do catch the same disease that one has. The illness in one can afflict the others. Sexual addiction might be a body disease that can spread to soul, and mind.

This way, lust was still at the age 59 writing lust infested checks that my means as well as my body could not possibly cash.

It seemed the more sexual pleasure I had, the hungrier I got for sex, and the more I wanted to have sex to make every moment of the short remaining part of my life to last.

These were some of the most intimate things that I had discussed with my therapist. This is what therapy is supposed to be. Unfortunately, some of the deep psychological wounds caused by sexual chronic depravation are difficult to deal with. When the urge or heat hits a man or a woman, all they can think of is how to get that sexual release and associated gratification. They want to be sexually satisfied and emotionally validated as a loving, caring, and sensual human with passion and burning desires. Most therapists try to reduce the boiling pleasure by trying to find something that went wrong somewhere during the patient's childhood and how to help the patient either forget, or under value, or just accept that he or she is not smart enough and that any such discussion with a therapist is inappropriate.

Then Hollywood does a somewhat of irresponsible act. It does objectify women, it does present a painted lady as what one has to have, and then bundles that with some hideous criminal or impossible situation. Therefore Hollywood is a giving a double message that sex is what we all need to have and we need to have saturated perfect sex with most beautifully painted partners.

Yet, after the sex drives hits a peak, then it routinely ignores, or cuts away from the scene. Imagine that you are hungry and thirsty. You go to a movie. For the first hour and a half, they show you the sexiest partners all painted and perfectly dressed and lighted. Then as you are dying to see more, the scene ends or something stupid happens and you never see the end of that scene.

After many therapy sessions, I had sort of figured it out. The Billion Dollar Madison Ave. advertising had brain washed me that at the end, the most important thing was to go to bed with one of the most beautiful women in the world.

I had just done that, but somehow, that had not quenched my thirst for intimacy, love, or even sex.

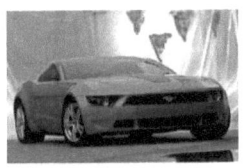 CHAPTER 3: Fire Engine Red Ford
Mustang and Fifth Ave. Roya Boutique

Roya subscribed to Bordeaux Fashion Journal which is similar to Elle Magazine, but it was even more elegant. Bordeaux also had patterns for the most attractive dresses attached to it. This magazine had the pictures of the most beautiful women in the world with the most beautiful and sexy dress and makeup.

These women were even more perfect than perfect! They all had an excellent make up that was just right and matched their skin complexion and dress color well. The choice of the dress was such to accentuate positive in their bodies and faces and minimize any imperfection. After all, all human beings do have some imperfection.

It was Roya's passion to decide which dress in each issue suited her best. She would then use the pattern to make her own dress. In most cases, these dresses made her just as attractive and sexy as the models that were on display in the Bordeaux Journal.

After our decision to get married, we two, like children who liked playing house, decided to select her dress and my tuxedo from fashion journals. I would daydream about going to parties or dancing with the best European clothes happily with family and friends. While sex had always meant a lot to me, sex was not the entire or the only thing. Fulfilling and satisfying sex was part of a loving marriage and a happy home.

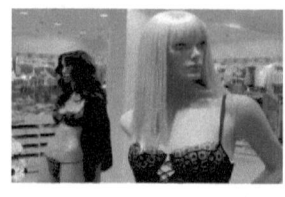 She had taught me a lot about the type of tuxedo that would look good on me. I have wide shoulders and my neck is just a bit too short. This meant that not every tuxedo would look nice on me. Keeping her suggestions in mind, we quickly selected the best tuxedo style for me. She had spent long time trying to figure out what looked best on her. She picked three final ones. We compared each one with the others carefully. She then turned to me and insisted to know what I thought. Blushing and being aroused at the same time, I told her that "Wedding ceremony will make me hot beyond any imagination. Naturally, right after the last guest had gone, my idea would be to have sex with you with the wedding dress still on!" Of course that wedding never took place.

It was not until many, many years later after Roya had broken up with me that I came across an elegant panties boutique right in the middle of Vienna Airport. Being essentially a reserved and shy person, it took me a few minutes to actually convince myself that I needed to see at least what they had. They had beautifully tailored panties from see-through fabric, also another fabric that felt and was colored just like Champaign and seemed to have some real gold strands in its fabric.

Suddenly, my eyes were fixated to their wedding collection. This was primarily because I had felt denied marrying Roya, and deprived forever of making passionate love to her. Most of the panties there were made from satin. Most seem to have a fascinating style. I asked the attractive and sexy saleswoman if I can touch the material. She was too quick to say "of course." Then she asked me if I was engaged. My immediate answer was, "Yes, I used to be! She is a sexy and beautiful half Persian and half French!" Then with a big regret I realized how much I missed her. I wish she was here with me.

The saleswoman, who was a tall, blonde, and sensuous woman in her thirties, got really interested. She asked, "What happened?" You are not engaged anymore?" I noticed that she was wearing a nicely cut skirt and a pair of nude colored stockings. As if to detract me from trying to mentally X-Ray her and see her nude body, she asked me, "How does this fabric feel?" One thing led to another, and I had to tell her that I only had a few quarters to live. "It is too bad! This is a shame! Life is short enough already. However, when people do not have a long time to live makes me really sad." The devil in me was cheering me to continue the "poor me, poor me" routine. This way I hoped this glamorous, irresistible, and hot woman feels sorry enough that she might go to bed with me to heal my wounds. This technique works well if the woman is hopelessly in a much higher league than I was in or even had any hopes to be in. She was just simply "too good for me!" Then she carefully studied my nice Nordstrom suit, my expensive briefcase, and my matching tie. Roya had trained me well when it came to organizing and selecting my outfits. Then, she carefully and slowly walked towards me in very small steps. I could tell that any surprise move from me would have scared and stopped her in her track completely since we were pure strangers. After all we had met only a few minutes prior to this. However we had met in a sexy place full of passion provoking panties.

As she got closer, I could see her cleavage. When she moved a bit closer and pretending to show me the other options, I noticed that her bra was made of lilac colored fabric. Then as our distance had shrunk to about less than one foot, I got a whiff of her scent. As I was trying to take a deep breath inhaling her scent, she whispered with a moaning and quietly asked, "Do you like my perfume? It is almost exactly what one of Mozart's lovers used to wear when they were young and crazy." Indeed, Austria and especially Vienna is all about Mozart. In Vienna you can find hundreds of different chocolate that is somehow named after Mozart. The same holds for Mozart drinks, foods and even T-shirts. It is no surprise that "Before Sunrise" movie which was a masterpiece regarding intimate and romantic relationships was entirely filmed there. Vienna served as that perfect background set for this elegant, romantic, and sexy movie.

While I was praying that she gets closer and closer to me so we can kiss or better yet, I can touch her under her hot panties, she seemed to focus on my fingers touching the crutch of one those wedding type panties. It seemed like I had turned into an ice statue with my two fingers touching the sizzling hot panties on the counter and my eyes were totally focused on her. This was all going on while I was bewildered, embarrassed, and explosively horny.

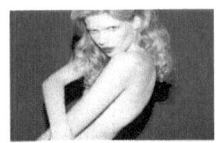

I was hot and my heart beat was twice the usual. Then, she stood on a small stepladder that had three steps. She did this so she can reach the panties that were on the top portion of the wall. "Sir, this one feels just like the one that you are touching right now. However, it is a bit more expensive because it has a nicely tailored opening in front. We custom make this so this opening is directly aligned and in front of a woman. This makes things easier during a moment of hot passion flare up. If you have the measurements, I can take it now and mail you the hand made one especially for your lover!" She did not seem to be scared of me after realizing up close that I had grayish silver hair and she had decided that I am a decent person. However, she did know for a fact that I was totally and painfully shy. I told her that I wished to touch that one too that was in the window. However, since I have a bad back, I cannot step on the ladder. "No problem Sir!" She flew down the steps of the ladder. Then my fantasizing and powerful imagination went into overdrive just like a 4 X 4 mussel truck goes into overdrive. I imagined that she had opened one of the drawers and took out a condom! "I was hot, I was delightful, and I was totally erected." She opened the lubricated condom packaging, and asked to see my fingers.

A few seconds passed by and I continued to be in mortal suspense. Then she took a casual look outside her store, and approached me. Sir, can you please put this condom on your two fingers. This was a delightful torture that was very sexy. After testing to make sure that the condom had gone as far up on my fingers as it could, she gently held my hand and motioned me to follow her as she went up the ladder. "Sir, since you cannot climb on the ladder, and since you asked how did the top panty felt, I like to let you feel it with your fingers. Better yet, I like to demonstrate it to you. But please do not get any wrong ideas in your head that I can see is throbbing with anticipation of sex!" My imagination as any dirty old man's imagination was flying in supersonic speeds.

By now, I could almost see her panties under her short skirt. At this point she poetically, moved my hand slightly closer to her panties. With her other hand, she gently lifted the skirt and gently slid my hand so my two fingers in the condom could touch her wet and hot pussy. I felt twenty years younger and full of sexual urge. My erection got even harder than I had ever felt before. She noticed my inhibition, so she decided to assure me that nobody could see what was happening. Then with her fingers she guided my two fingers close to her soft, supple, shaved, and erotic pussy. I was had! I did not care about the announcement about my Austrian Airline's final boarding. All I could think about was how her pussy would feel if she let me insert my two fingers in. Surprise, before I knew it, my two fingers inside the condom were completely inside her. She was quietly moaning and saying things in her native language that I could not understand. She was really wet and hot and she was so ever gently vibrating forward and backward.

I had no problem finding her clit. Then as if I had made a discovery, "Oh, you are wearing a tampon, I hope that I did not hurt you." Her answer was swift. Then in a feminine voice she encouraged and pleaded with me to please, please finish her up. I started to move my fingers sideways and search for her clit again. Then with ever so loving voice, she would guide me where to go and what to do. "Left, more left, please touch the wall! Now right. Now, please go deeper, and deeper. Faster, and then suddenly stop or go to the other side." Then all of sudden looking like a professor, "Now let me teach you something that American women do not know. Here, please spread your fingers to open me as wide as you possibly can. It is OK. This does not hurt. Remember that two full term babies have come out from there. It was a big pleasure. See, it stretches and you can not hurt it."

Once she was done with her instructions, she took her fingers and quickly unrolled the condom and pulled it off my fingers. "Here, spread my pussy as much as you can again. It can easily stretch about six Centimeters (which is about two Inches)". Then something happened that I had never seen before in my life. This happened a few minutes after she had ordered me to do an in and out motion! Then, "watch, please watch." Followed by, "I will come in three seconds!"
Before it had taken those three seconds, a tiny bit of fluid gushed out of her pussy and splashed on my face and shirt. The fluid had the consistency of very light nonfat milk mixed with naturally lubricated water and it had no smell. It was delightfully warm. "Did you ever see a woman have such strong orgasm and come so big? This is my come and I am mighty proud of it."
Then, as if something terrible had happened, she informed me that my flight had departed 10 minutes ago. Then she gave me an interesting offer. You can wait for the next flight that will be in two hours, or stay with me tonight and then I promise you to bring you back to the airport in time before the first flight to New York tomorrow.
I was standing right next to her and daydreaming about fantastic sex with her. I am sure that she could easily read my naughty mind on what my preference was.
We got to her nice and roomy apartment in less than twenty minutes. Then we both took shower together. She seemed to get another orgasm by opening her vagina and letting water from the shower wash over it. She still had some of her ejaculation left. I was uncontrollably horny, so I had to again feel her. When I inserted my fingers in, I noticed that she was still very soft and warmly lubricated.

As we were approaching her bed, she had a belt and a hand cuff along with a golden dildo. Apologizing as hard as I could, I told her that I am sorry, but I cannot deal with these things. I do not like them and I have never had these and will never have them. Her honest reaction was, "No worries, I just want to show you an excellent time!" Then after puckering her beautiful lips that were covered in black lipstick she seemed to ask me for a kiss.

A confession just had to come. I told her, "I am sorry, I cannot deal with black lipstick either. It turns me off. I am sorry." She used some of the cosmetic removal wet towels from her pocket and demanded to know what color of lipstick would turn me on. "Something that is light chocolate, has a little of bronze, and is crisp and soft. Oh, I also love lip plumpers."

Then, suddenly I got extremely upset. Somehow it felt like I had woken up in the middle of a nice dream. I looked around, and I was still in that panties shop and I was dying with desire to act out in real life what I must have been imagining in a wet dream kind of daydream. This mostly happens when one is sleep and the sleep is somehow disrupted. One wakes up, stays sort of awake for a few seconds or minutes, and then resumes deep sleep quickly. This was happening to me. It was happening in real life, in real daylight, in an international airport and right in the presence of the sexiest woman in the world that was that saleswoman. It was even stronger than that, she was standing right next to me. She had an inviting smile on her beautiful face that somehow was telling me that she could easily be reading my mind, and vividly watching, with me and seeing my daydream. This is very similar to satisfied feeling that two lovers get watching TV after an entire night of heavy lovemaking.

No sooner had I gotten back to sleep - I mean strong daydreaming – that I seemed to see the rest of the erotic movie in my mind. I saw her say, "Let us get into the bed." Then after a minute of hesitation she added, "Would you like me to get on the top since you have a bad back?" I said no problem at all. She was on top pumping and riding me as fast as she could. "Man you are as hard as a rock!" Then she reached my lips and gave me kisses while I was in her. After some of the sexiest kisses that I have ever experienced, then she lifted her shoulders by leveraging her hands. This way she could slap my face with her gentle, beautiful, and soft breasts by making sharp side by side motion on her upper body. It took some time for me to learn to enjoy both of these motions that were going on at the same time. I really enjoyed this.

Then we decided to get our sleep since we both were working the next day. Of course, my work was on board the long flight and I had to prepare statistics about last year's expenses and profits.

In my dream, I started to see sexy women touching me. I was dreaming that I was standing on top of a nice high mountain that was higher than clouds and was having standing sex with an attractive TWA flight attendant. As if this was not enough, I dreamed that next day we were in one of those hidden beds somewhere in the middle of their planes but away from the passenger's eyes. The dream was too exciting and I woke up. I saw her giving me oral sex. I had a condom on and that was smeared with her beautiful chocolate bronze lipstick. I was not fully awake after she asked me if I wanted to penetrate her pussy. She then added, "Honey, you were too excited to go to deep sleep. Your entire 16 Centimeter (about 7 1/2 Inches) penis was fully erect. It was so rock hard that it was trying to go right into her thy like a knife." She got on top of me and repeated the "Push, Push, In and Out, and breast slaps sideways." When she announced a break, I was kissing her on the neck and pussy. This is when she decided to give me some of the best French kisses that I have ever had in my entire life up to that point.

I came! In fact it was a big burst even though there was not enough to ejaculate like the last time.

As my luck would have it, my back started to experience a great deal of pain! I thought that I will die. In fact, I knew that I really deserved to die. I had had three or four times more sex in one session that I had ever had before."

She went into a feeling of sorrow and remorse. "This is entirely my fault. I acted like a whore, and a demanding whore at that!" "I am sorry, can you forgive me?" Then she added, "I am sorry. I knew that Americans are not as spontaneous and passionate as we Europeans. I am sorry."

"No, no, no, please do not blame this on yourself!" I said emphatically.

"OK, then let me take care of you. I had one year of nursing school before my husband at the time nagged me to stop the school and start working full time." Moments later we were facing each other in the bed. I gently pushed my own thy up in between her perfumed and supple legs and moved it so I can touch and feel her burning pussy. Her pussy had become a hot oven by then."

"I know that you admired my long fingers. I am cupping my fingers on both bands so you can snuggly put your beautiful, long, and thick penis in my cupped hands." Then, while she was holding my penis with one cupped hand, she gently put both balls in her other hand by gently pushing the other hand underneath them. This gave me a feeling that I will never forget. I had barely felt sleep again when I turned around and my penis had left her cupped fingers. I was daydreaming that I was sleep and in bed with one of the worlds most sexy and beautiful women.

When I woke up a few minutes later, I saw her applying some lipstick to the inseam of one those white satin panties. Then she sprayed a little Chanel Number 5 right on the crutch and used this panty to almost cover the lamp shade while exuding a sexy aroma. In a few minutes the scent of Chanel 5 along with the scent of that Milani lipstick had turned that room into a heaven.

I felt that she sprayed something on my penis. I knew that she would not hurt me. "What is this spray?" She assured me by saying, "You will know it in a few minutes." Sure enough in a few minutes I was completely erect. This would have been my third intercourse in less than six hours. I was absolutely sure that I had no more fluid left to come again. She was kissing me and fondling my penis. Then as she was excitedly looking at my penis, she said, "Man you are lucky. You are beefy and thick and long. I love it when your penis reaches and touches my clit." Then taking a sip of her Cognac, she encouraged me to drink mine. I had to say, "I am sorry, I do not drink!"

A little later, I heard the sound of boiling water in the kitchen. She then rushed to the kitchen and removed the kettle from the oven. The next thing I heard was the sound of ice cubes crashing as they were being emptied in a bowl. She then entered the room with ice bowl in one hand and hot water in the other. By then my erection was so hard that I could not sit comfortably if I wanted to. In addition, the fact that she was totally nude and only wearing a trace amount of Coco perfume seemed to make me even more fiercely excited.

"I will take good care of you! Please turn on your belly." She gently and carefully was putting hot and cold compress on my lower back while her supple and shaved pussy was in contact with my buns or the back of my leg or thy. My back was feeling great, so I asked her if I can turn around. As I was half way turning I noticed that my penis had never, ever been that big ever before. In fact being on the bed face down was painful since my penis was so long and so solid that it seemed like I had to turn around or it would break! It was that hard.

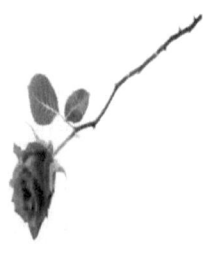

A more careful and delightful observation of my penis showed that it was covered by a color that was very similar to Nordstrom's "Red Army" colored lipstick. She had applied that to my entire penis. My balls were perfectly covered. My penis shaft was completely covered. Then I delightfully noticed that my entire penis was shaved. There was no hair to see anywhere. I, along with my penis could be aroused with the slightest of air movement in the apartment. This is what lipstick applied on penis does. The lipstick would give a cool feeling and at the same time add to friction that creates more sexual enjoyment. Another side effect is that in a few days after this the penis feels extremely supple and soft.

"I want to give you another pleasure before we go our separate ways. Remember after we each will go our ways, God only knows when we will see each other again! So, we have this night and let us make the best out of it. For all I know, we might not even be alive tomorrow or the next day." As per her instructions, I was on my back again with a fully erected penis that seemed to reach the ceiling, and she was telling me to spread my legs just a bit more. Then she delightfully announced, "Fine, fine keep it that way." Then with her back towards me, she mounted on top of me and holding my penis with two fingers. Then she lowered her body slowly so my penis would delightfully penetrate her really hot and already pulsating and quivering pussy." This time just like a jockey that was riding a horse, she was riding me, or more precisely, my fully erected penis.

I noticed that although she had carefully covered my penis with lipstick, I had no condom on. She noticed my alarm and assured me that it is OK since she was wearing a female condom. I had never seen a female condom before and I did not see it that night either as we went at having sex for a few hours. I started to feel spasms that felt like I was getting ready to come, or die, or both. Being trained as a nurse, she must have sensed this, but she pretended to ignore it. Then she informed me, "Honey you have nothing left to come; just enjoy the sex."

We both fell asleep hugging each other with our lips caressing. Six o'clock in the morning arrived much sooner than I had thought. I could not leave her after this loving and sexually ultimate experience. I had to get more, and more, and if it killed me, then so be it.

She was serving breakfast before I knew it. There were three different cheeses and four different chocolates along with a steaming hot cup of chocolate. I first managed to drink up all the regular and mineral water that was on my side, and even drink those that were on her side as soon as she had offered them to me. I was delightfully feeling dehydrated after intense sex orgy that we had had.

Much to my disbelief, right after having our breakfast, she was on her knees under the table giving me the best oral sex that I had ever had. I was again unprotected, but she had covered the inside of her mount with a generous portion of saran wrap. Somehow she went out of control, and spitted the saran wrap out and went full blast on giving me a superb blow job. This time after I had slept a few hours, to my amazement, I was ejaculating and ejaculating heavy right in her beautiful mouth. Her tongue had quickly learned how to whirl around my penis so we both enjoy a great deal of sexual pleasure.

I did not have to insist when I suggested that we regroup in my hotel room that had a beautiful view. She quickly put her stuff in her overnight bag and we were on our way. My hotel room with all upgrades that I could squeeze out of my United Airlines Frequent Flyer was right next to the swimming pool.

She had called in sick and I had just simply asked to take a day of vacation. This hotel mainly catered to the business people who were on company paid business trips. So, it seemed to be deserted around 10:00 AM when we arrived since most businessmen had to go work at that hour.

We then went swimming right away. I had lost some weight and my swimming trunk was somewhat puffy and loose on me. "Honey, you are still excited! Let me service you!" Before I knew, my beige swimming trunk was lowered by her since he had dived into the water. I looked up and there was an older man sitting in a balcony enjoying his early lunch and carefully observing us. I think that she too knew this perfectly well. But he pretended that he was not watching us. However, I knew that he was watching us all the time even when he would pretend that he is watching the other side. My partner, being worried that we might be detected, speeded up her movements back and forth with her tongue on my penis.

A bartender then showed up. I pushed my partner up. She being smart knew that something had happened. She came up right away. She ordered her favorite Cognac and hot steaming milk for me. While I seemed to be somewhat ashamed of what we were doing right in the open and day light, my partner was literally high and was savoring every minute of it. As our drinks were delivered, there seemed to be a quick exchange of very polite words between my sexual partner and the bartender. They both seemed to agree and the bartender left. Even though I speak four languages I was not able to really understand what they said to each other.

About ten minutes later after we had leisurely sipped most of our drinks, my sexual partner asked me to please close my eyes. I totally surrendered without any hesitation. Soon, I felt something very soft covering my left toe while other toes, were touching what must have been a woman's soft body. "Please keep your eyes shut, you will really like this." I obeyed without any resistance. Then I felt the other toe touching another soft body. While I was getting used to this sensation, my toe was guided to push into some soft velvet material and get into a warm pussy. In fact a few seconds after my toe penetrated, I felt a strong pulsing and palpitation along with warm fluid. She was ejaculating and I was happy and proud of that.

Since, I was sitting on the steps and was covered by water just only to my belt level; I felt being kissed by two hot lips at the same time and on my lip with one on each side. In a few seconds after their tongue had been poetically yet passionately touched under my tongue and the inside of my lips, I was able to taste a faint taste of a sweet liquor on one, and on the other, a bittersweet yet very fancy tropical fruit. I was being French kissed by two very powerful yet very soft tongues penetrating each side of my mouth. This was the same two lovely women who were pushing my toes into their pussies under the water. These were the two friends of my original partner. My toe was penetrated their pussies and they were French kissing me. Oops, there was another. This was my original sexual partner from the panty shop. She was giving me oral sex under the water and coming up to breath air and then would go down again on my penis. "I am honestly obsessed with your penis, you, and your American ways of doing things. Also, I find you very desirable and sexy with your silver hair and hazel eyes. You are clean, patient, and considerate.

By now the old man was too horny to continue eating his lunch in the balcony and he was totally absorbed in watching us. I started to worry that he might have a heart attack and fall down! Right about then I felt something soft being rubbed on my penis under the water. My sexual partner had asked one of the two girls to give her the chocolate pudding that she did not feel like eating. Since it had come from refrigerator, it was still cold. The pride was getting to my head and I was having the sex of my lifetime. She loved my penis more than her favorite chocolate pudding. Soon, while the two women were using my toes as a dildo and were getting ready to come, I felt my penis in my partner's mouth that was full of chocolate pudding. In less than 20 seconds of her licking and sucking on my penis with the chocolate pudding, I came so hard that I begin to see stars. After taking a few more minutes with the other toe in the other women, she started to come as a result of having "Toe Sex" with me.

Most of this was going on before the sunrise even though it had gone on for some time. We felt some privacy as long as those megawatt swimming pool lights had not been lit.

My heart beat was approaching twice its normal rate. I was in heavens. I was trembling with excitement. My body and soul was resonating with each and every ejaculation of others and myself.

All of a sudden there seemed to be a lot of light!

I quickly pulled out both toes. Then, I pushed my original lover gently away. The double French kiss that they were giving me stopped and the two lovely ladies kissed me on the chick and disappeared in a fast dash. It was only after noticing that they had left that I began to get sad for their disappearance. I was happy to see that the light that was coming was not from the swimming pool lights. It was from one of the luxury rooms directly across from us. As I looked closer, I noticed a very attractive woman, in very thin lingerie sitting on a chair looking outside. Come to think of it, I am positive that she must have sat there for some time and watched us. The lingerie, that I could guess must come from some of the most famous Paris galleries, was tan in color and it was basically see through.

In a blink of the eye, she opened her glass sliding door and dived into the pool from other side. She swam under the water for the most of time coming directly towards my erected penis. As she was pulling that beautiful and perfectly sexy body out the water, her thin panties started to slide own on her thighs and soon, she was completely nude waist down. She was perfectly shaved and her pussy, that she proudly called her cunt, was shinning just like a mirror.

By then, she had gotten to my side of the swimming pool with her hotly desirable body and cunt. She gently stopped behind me so the back of my head could feel the heat of her hot cunt! In my ears, the word cunt is even more powerful than any aphrodisiacs imaginable. Seconds after this, I felt the tip of her tongue magically and rhythmically bring my fact, and my entire being to boiling temperature. The scent of her lilac and jasmine perfume mixed with chlorine from the swimming pool had just made things more and more intensive. Nevertheless, she was one of those women who had colder body temperature compared to those who have higher. In general, I always prefer those who have cooler temperature. I do not want fire to blaze from two heated bodies if we go to bed together. I was going crazy with the scent, and her unbelievable beauty, style, and movements. They were so poetic and gentle that I could not wait any longer. Just about the time that her piano-player long fingers were finding their way under my erected penis and were gently teasing my balls, I had realized that if all other girls were sex artists, this lady must be the top and best of all. Then just as gently, she swiftly but lovingly cupped her long fingers around my penis so I can feel her touch with the top of my scrotum. Then she so ever gently touched by the middle of the palm of her hand. She was gentle and caring. It truly felt the type of touching that goes on between honeymooners that were deeply in love.

Then, she moved the palm of her hand slightly so the only point of contact be right between the sulcus part corona on the top and her very supple skin. I was extremely hot. She confidently and erratically begged, "Stop these motions to prolong my sexual pleasure." The tip of her tongue was touching my forehead so gently, that I did not know if this was my imagination or her tongue. Her tongue patiently yet carefully travelled down my face. From forehead, the tip of her tongue was caressing to top of my nose, then upper lip and then one of the most heavenly French kiss. She did all of this standing directly over my head while the back of my head was touching her pussy. By then I started to feel her excited and beautiful nipples on the sides of my head going down towards my face.

I was bursting with sizzling heat, when I heard an observation from this woman. "Oh my God help me. Look at that fully erected and beautiful penis!" I had just detected a slight Scandinavian accent when she said, "Can you bone me! Can you please let me come? I have been watching you all this time this afternoon or evening from behind our window and with all lights shut off so you could not see."

"Do you like my cunt as much as I like your penis?" Suddenly swimming pool lights came on. We all ran for shelter. It was not just the swimming pool; it was also the balcony lights and many other outdoor lights. Much to our relief no one else was watching and there were no guards telling us to leave. She then pleaded with me and my partner to go join her and her husband for a final course in their room."

We had to oblige, you cannot say no to a sexy Norwegian. Another forty-five minutes went by while we were busy on a foursome. Once this was done, those who still had some come left got the last bit of or their come out and just like athletics after a major game, one by one fell asleep.

After the heavy sex was completed this time, and when her pussy was right in front of my face I kissed it. Then, I rubbed my face in this beautiful pussy before my right hand came up to touch her. "Please, please. I need more. I am not quite satisfied after all these. Please, please."

Then all three came up and we all hugged. Somehow the old man watching us was an irresistible aphrodisiac for all three women. My original sexual partner seemed to be finally completely satisfied.

Then, one of the women asked something in a whispering voice from my original partner. She immediately asked me, "Honey, they want you to push your beautiful penis into each of their pussies one at a time. They will not take off their bikinis so the old man upstairs will not know. They will French kiss you and have sex with you under the water at the same time until you cannot do it anymore. Just about the time I was done asking "Condoms, how about any protection?" I was having heavy sex with one of the woman who had short blonde hair. My penis had penetrated her as if they know each other for years and years. It seemed like my penis was thinking and acting on its own and totally independent of me. By now, my toe was still inside the other woman who was a bit older and with brunette hair. I noticed the blonde woman was really a natural blonde. Her eye brows were blonde and more importantly all her pubic her was a beautiful soft silky blonde. She was very gentle with my penis. In a few minutes after this, I felt she was coming on my penis. I could not possibly come, but she was elated with her overactive pulsating clit to have had double orgasm. By now, my stupid committee was shaming me. "Hey, are you a production horse? Why are these women so interested and excited by you? Where is the fine print? What will they give you? I mean AIDS, or what?"

As the second woman had had her fill, she slowly pushed aside and gave me a kiss and a hug. Then she went down in the water and brushed her completely natural and gorgeous blonde hair against my left thy and then more forcefully brushed it again my penis. This hair brush was exactly what I needed to regain my erection for the final sexual act. The brunette lady had smaller breasts, but her pussy was nicely shaped and very juicy.

Suddenly, I heard somebody clapping. The clapping was not too loud, but it was intended for four of us to hear! It was the old man. "Bravo! The best fireworks I have ever seen!" I am young again and I want to make love! Then as if worried to have created a scene he sat down on his chair. However, he could not finish his lunch. He was watching a world-class performance from the balcony of his hotel room.

The brunette was asking me if I was tired. She was touching me under the water. Then my original partner told her something. She got out of the pool and went to the table nearby to get her hand bag. She came back with some blush and a blush brush, foundation powder, and a really nice lipstick that was wine colored and matched her sexy hair perfectly. "Your friend tells me watching a woman put on this particular makeup turns you on! Let me see if it works." She applied this makeup the same way an artist uses a paint brush to create a master piece of beauty on canvas. Then another quick word and the brunette dived down to apply the lipstick on my penis.

When the soft tip of lipstick gently rubs on my penis, the result is always magical and instant. It is a big hard on. Just a few seconds after I was hard enough, my penis was sliding into her just the same way that lipstick glides and smoothly goes into a lipstick cover.

Unlike the softness that I have enjoyed with the blonde, the brunette was passionate. Her back and forth motion was creating bubbles, circles looking like tiny whirlpools, and a swishing sound in the swimming pool water. Then she pushed me down one more step and asked me to please spread my legs so that she can get more penetration. A few more strong back and forth and ins and outs she had her first strong orgasm. Her vibrating vagina started to spew hot soup all around my penis. The soup was so thick that I could see some of it as it came out of her and into the swimming pool water. Of course, her come would dissolve quickly.

Just about the time that I was happy that I had served these two women and they have served me the best way possible, I felt something hot and burning coming out of my penis. It was a fluid and thanks God, it was not blood. What was going on? It must have been the heat in her vagina combined with her hot and acidic ejaculation had started to cause that burning sensation. Of course, by then I had had hours of sex. In fact we all had had sex for too many hours for me to remember. The brunette was now begging me. "Please, please let me come a second time. I am almost there and it will be a big one. Please be patient with me."

I noticed that the bra support behind her was broken and now her beautiful tiny breasts with an eighth of an inch long erected nipples were also brushing against my chest. "Wait, wait, wait honey, let me kiss you. I need that before I can manage to come! Please let me be completely satisfied." She then proceeded to give me two or three more French kisses with her unusually long tongue and then gently touch the tip of my tongue with the top of hers. She was kissing me and was masturbating me at the same time with her shapely hands.

I started to feel an urge to come, so I entered her again. It seemed like the miracle had happened and I would come again. She was passionately having sex with me, and then we both came at the same time. When we were ejaculating at the same time, I continued to feel the burning sensation. For a few seconds, I would feel the burning hot come from her to be mixed and cooled down with my cooler come. She gave out a loud joyful scream. Then she was so relaxed that she seemed to fall asleep.

Shortly after this, I felt a sexy touch in my ear. It was the one to my right. She was asking for a Vanilla Chocolate Swirl. The blonde, ultra sexy, and gracions blonde said, S'il vous plaît, monsieur me donner un tourbillon de chocolat et de vanille, s'il vous plaît.

Some men are proud of driving a 4 X 4 big truck (Four by four, which means that that truck or car is so powerful that all 4 tires have drive power as opposed to normal cars that have only 2 tires with the drive power). Having completed this sex act, this act that almost cost my life, now in Madam François's elite and distinctive club; I had qualified for the 1 X 6 (One by Six which means one man and six woman instantly having sex at the same time) certification!

This is a sensation overload that gives a man as much of sexual pleasure, all at the same time, as possible. At first my mind was trying to feel each sexual partner's touch and feel one at a time. Then, and quickly, my mind decided to cherish and rejoice and take as much as possible all at the same time. I was feeling those feelings everywhere. Subconsciously, I knew that I had never had this massive luxury, nevertheless, I wanted more and more!

Without much effort, I remembered that Chocolate Vanilla Swirl was a soft serve ice cream where these two flavors were mixed together in a corkscrew action. Triumphantly, I realized that that blonde wanted me to turn my fingers that were happily enjoying being into her in a cork screw action. I was elated to oblige. In fact I would have obliged and done anything for such a blonde beauty even if my life depended on it.

Right at that moment, I seemed to have blacked out. The interesting thing was that the last time that I had blacked out was some twenty years prior to this. That black out was induced with cheap fraternity bear and excessive drinking. Somehow, I was trying to open my eyes a bit wider so I can maybe see again. Unfortunately this was not working. I was going to scream for help but I just could not. Then, I felt that my heart was beating very fast, and then it felt like it stopped all together. There was a feeling of weightlessness and euphoria as if I had died. This is what is called sudden death as a result of massive amounts of sex overdose!

As I seemed to momentarily come to after that almost sudden death, I quickly helped the brunette tie her bra strips behind her. She helped me pull up my swimming trunk. By then it was about 2:00 PM. We retired to a table nearby to order lunch. By now the old man had come downstairs to join us for lunch. Without any hesitation, we all agreed. The old guy was a retired SAS, the Scandinavian Airline pilot. He was about 71 and was visiting his grand kids here in Vienna.

I know that you all think that this must have been a wet dream of mine, a fantasy that can only happen in a dream. You might be right. However, in this perfect fantasized dream, this was the graduating class of Madam François. Depending on how good they were in having sex with a total stranger, they each got a grade. Madam Francois only graduated and hired the best of the best. In this case, I was the unsuspecting total stranger.

We could see that this old man was horny as hell. The brunette who was not completely satisfied even after coming twice started some small talk with him. The old man spoke her language fluently. Then I passed out again. When I came to this time, I noticed that the brunette went under the table, and opened the old man's zipper and started to give him a slow blow job. The old man was in heavens.

My sudden death had persisted for a few seconds, minutes, or even hours as I was concerned, when I came to for just a few instants.

During those instants, I could see Madam François desperately, yet professionally giving me mouth to mouth resuscitation. Then, I could barely remember being in an ambulance on the way to Emergency Room at some Vienna hospital. In addition, she sat right next to my bed in Emergency Room up until I was given permission to go home. Of course, home in this case meant my hotel room.

Madam François walked and talked just like Kat in Sherry's Ranch. They both are professional, caring, sexy, and responsible at the same time. Kat drinks only coffee and she always gives a big hug afterwards. In her profile in Sherry's Ranch, she says that she speaks two languages fluently. These two languages are English and Spanish. Then for Spanish, she adds that Spanish is the language of love. It is interesting that language or act of physical love and love making seem to blur when I was making love to her, or just having pure and unattached sex. For an irresistibly sexy woman to feel and act this way, it is phenomenal.

The fantasy wet dream ended as I paid for the panties that I had purchased and left that store and re-entered the real world with all its dull life. But, was it completely a dream, a sexy flight of fancy? This thought echoed what I had heard from TJ, that superb blonde that I had met at Sherry's Ranch in Pahrump, Nevada near Las Vegas. Of course, Sherry's Ranch is a legal and premier American brothel. TJ had told me, "Bryce, sex is mostly in your head. While there are heavy physical aspects to it, the biggest part of the pleasure comes from your thoughts. The fact is that physical tender touch and intimacy helps expedite and magnifies those feelings and sensations.

The next day as I was getting started to board my flight back home, I felt like I had to go to that panty shop. I had no name, I had no telephone number, and I had no contact information. However, I easily found it as it was near my departure gate. The saleswoman, who was working there this day, had a very strong East European accent and she seemed to not be interested even in talking to me. Quite contrary to the beautiful and feminine one that had met me before, this woman was heavy set and looked somewhat manly. "Sir, please make your selection. Then let me know and I will ring you up quickly. Before you ask, let me tell you that you cannot touch the material that my panty is made of and I am wearing right now. Also, let me tell you that you cannot ask me to model those split in front panties for you. I am happily married to a really strong man and we make love at least once a day!" Then as an afterthought, she added that she would not give her panties to anyone so they can feel it and touch the heat in the crutch. She was serious and I could tell that she really meant what she was saying.

For whatever reason, with all the harsh words, she retrenched a bit later on and felt somewhat sorry for me. She said "The woman, who dived into the swimming pool, was a graduate of Madam François and she was assigned to test the latest graduates. You must feel bad that you were the test target. However, you can be with any of them if you like. It will cost somewhere from $400 to $800/Hr. However, they are all a steal at this price because they can make you the happiest and most satisfied man on earth! Would you like their phone numbers?" Was I imagining again?

I boarded my flight with somewhat of bitterness and sadness like a spoiled kid who demanded, and felt entitled to the same amount of heavy sex every day as if sex was like a kid's toy. As my Austrian Airlines flight took off, I started to think back about Roya. I remembered how important it was for us and our families to be proper and conform to all strict standards at the time. We had not had any sex ever in our lives. However, to play by the book and be good citizens, we were going to have sex only after marriage. However, right after all the sex that I have had, I still yearn for what it would have been if I had married Roya when we were both virgins. The idea of having sex once and perhaps last time a few instants before officially being married was conceptually OK with her. Before she could say anything, I could see that she too was blushing. Then being a man and a very hot and excited man right at that moment, I told her, "Let us go and get our virginity out of the way, now. I cannot wait!"

Roya took all of that in and then said "My parents have been dreaming about this marriage all their lives. Let us do the honorable thing and not break their hearts!" After a short pause, she continued, "If you wait, then I promise to have sex with you with wedding dress on, in the fire engine red Ford Mustang and in my boutique in the Fifth Ave. But since Roya Boutique will be an official business, we can have sex before opening, or after closing."

For many years, I have wondered what Roya would have felt if she was standing on one of the balconies watching just like the old man did. Then the next natural question is would I have done all this sex if I was happily and sexually satisfied if I had been married to Roya? This would have been the case, especially if we had had two kids and a loving marriage. Maybe not and maybe yes. I will never know that for the life of me.

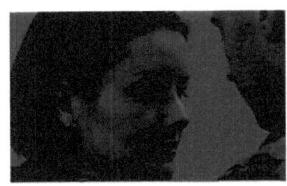 CHAPTER 4: The First, First Love's Goodbye

During the last time that I met Roya for a goodbye, she told me that her dad had promised to get her wedding dress from Gallery La Fayette in Paris. These stores are like our Nordstrom. The one in Paris has seven floors with a restaurant on the seventh floor with a breath taking view of Paris.

She then stopped talking abruptly. Then she tried to wipe off a tear that had started to come down her eyes. Then, suddenly as if not being able to stop a storm, tears raced down her eyes nonstop.

"Why is this happening to us?" "Is God this merciless?" Then she put her head on my shoulder and cried. Then, she raised her head just a bit and asked again "Why, Why?"

The waitress, who had just taken the first hastened step to come to our table, made a quick U turn and went to anther table to let us catch our breath.

I was numb. I did not really know what to say.

This had hit me just as unexpectedly and painfully as it had hit her. Unfortunately being a man, society expected me to be emotionless and macho. Hell, I did play the part, but when I got home I was crying just as hard.

It was very nice of Roya to say goodbye. It was the ethical and honorable thing to do. She was not able to give me any reason for why this had happened. She was just as lost as I was.

Sometimes I think that we might have been absolutely miserable if we had married. Sometimes, I think that there must have been some heavenly reason why our marriage did not happen.

But who knew, we could also have been madly in love and happily married after all these years.

My wife has always had an interesting theory about her and me. Her theory is that we should have never, ever been married! "Look there is nothing in this marriage! We do not talk, we have no sex, we have no intimacy, we have no money, and we have no future!" Then just the same way that an attorney breathes a sigh of relief after a convincing and earth shattering argumentation, my wife took a deep breath and said "Let us file for a divorce!"

Then she triumphantly walked towards the refrigerator, found some old containers with peanut butter, Jelly, and a bottle of flat Coke. She sat at the table ready to make her sandwich. Before she could say anything, I jumped and did the gallant thing and gave her a loaf of bread. She was going to say thanks. But she stopped right in the middle and then went back to saying "Were you listening to me?"

This I was convinced would have never, ever happened with Roya!

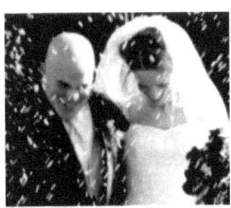

CHAPTER 5: Pete's Marriage

Pete is almost like a brother to me. We went to graduate school together and he has always been my pillar of strength. He seemed to always be there to hear my side of the story. He was nonjudgmental; he was always ready to help.

I had told him my story of Roya and he was able to help me understand that sometimes life does not turn out to be what we like. His family being from main land China, and from a socialite and wealthy had always provided him with the best. Pete and his family would go to winter ski trips to Zermatt in Switzerland, and Banff resorts in Canada that was pre-planned and annual. When Pete was six his family noticed that he was attached to her niece. They seem to like to do everything together. So, in the grand authentic Chinese tradition his father and Lucy's father "promised" these two together.

They were sweethearts for many years. Unfortunately, around high school these loved ones decided that the promise will not work for them.

Pete started to look around. He was determined to be happily married to a good Chinese woman. He almost got married to an American but then things did not work and the engagement broke. It seemed that like me, he was held back because of a dream. This was a daydream just like my constant Roya dreams.

Pete helped me get a good job with a major corporation and relocate to California to live near San Francisco. We had rejoined after several years. Just like college days, we started to double date. But neither of us was overly excited or eager.

One day, Pete told me that he had a plan. He really wanted a Chinese wife. Therefore, it made sense that he went where there were a lot of Chinese. That meant that he would go to the local college that taught Chinese. His strategy was to take a class pretending that he did not know any Chinese. The fact remained that he was fluent in Chinese.

He soon became the star student who helped everyone with their home work. He got a lot of attention from everyone. There were several strikingly attractive Chinese women. He had even dated two of them. One day he told me that he is tired. He has had enough of this single life. He wants a true love, he wants to settle down. "Pete, for most of your life, and mine for that matter, we have been sort of like Playboys. We have always been in hot pursuit of one woman or the other. How could you get tired?" "I do not know!" he confessed. However, he added that when was listening to "Just Call Me an Angle in the Morning" song something had happened to him.

He felt a cold feeling that even though he was over-sexed, he was awfully under-loved.

As legends would have it, he fell in love with one girl in the class who had a deformed nose. He had had coffee with her at the beginning of the semester. Nevertheless the relationship quickly rekindled itself after they decided to write the final essay for the class together.

"But Pete you told me that Sylvia's deformed nose was a turn off! You told me that she did not know how to dress. You told me that she wore almost no makeup." "Bryce, that was before my epiphany. I am in love!" "I have found the love of my life." "I have found my forever!"

He convinced Sylvia to care for herself more and get the surgery she needed to open the air passage in her nose. Coming out of that surgery that had an additional part to make her nose look better, she told Pete that this is what she should have done many years ago.

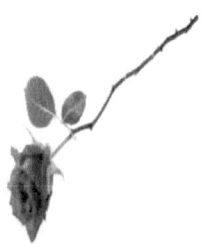

My entire family and I were invited to a fantastic Chinese wedding in Chicago.

Pete and Sylvia have moved back to Chicago and they have three wonderful boys. In a recent trip to Chicago, I caught up with Pete and Sylvia. After a nice home-made lunch, we went for our long walk together.

I had prepared myself to hear some stuff about affairs, or some other things from the playboy that Pete used to be. "No, I gave all of that up!" He added, "Do not get me wrong, I do not have a perfect marriage. But somehow it seems that she fulfills me and completes my life."

Pete had told me one day that just like Dean Martin who was Jerry Louise's comedy partner; he always thought that the next woman that he would "bed down" will give him that perfect sex. Just like the alcoholic who thinks the next drink will finally quench his thirst.

Just like Dean, Pete would look at a pretty woman and could not wait until he found what kind of panties she had on. Or, it could be even more enticing if she had no panties on. As my buddy of all these years, he had confided in me that he can pretty much tell what brand of panties a particular woman wore.

In fact, he had gotten so good at this that this panty conversation was his pick up line when he first met women. I remember one night he ordered a drink for a woman across the bar who was not returning his eye contact. Then, he moved to sit near her with the middle seat empty. This time, he succeeded in starting a conversation. Soon the panty question came up. "I think that as an attractive, warm, and cultured woman, you must like to wear Olga brand panties!" She cuddled her drink for a few long seconds. Then she started to say something, but she stopped before the first word came up.

After finishing her drink and a few minutes before closing of the bar, she cleared her throat and told him in whispering yet horny voice, "Yes I wear Olga brand panties. I will let you cream my hot one that I am wearing now. Are you man enough to take me to a nice hotel, and cream my Olga panties?"

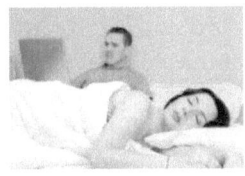 CHAPTER 6: Sex Deprived, Sex Crazed, Sexual Depression, and Sexual Addiction

I just had to call my buddy of all these years and tell him what was happening to me. We had always shared our experiences even when we felt stupid or worried.

"Pete, I am scared and I am worried." He jokingly asked me if I had the "Laptop" problem again. This was a code word between him and me so our wives could not figure out what we talking about. Laptop to me meant asking a lover sit on my lap to share some tender moments. Of course, a laptop to our wives had the innocent sound of a computer laptop.

"No Pete and I do not feel like joking. Sorry." Inquisitively, but caringly, he said "Tell me what is on your mind. We always did all these years." I almost did not say it, but too late the words had come out of my mind. "Pete, I am dying. Like an old car, I am falling apart. It seems like a piece of me dies more and more each day. I am not used to this." "I cannot keep it up long enough to be good in bed. The surgeon says that I need to get a cadaver disk to replace my broken one in my lower back." All hell broke loose. I could hear Peter's screams saying "Do not do it!" "I did it and I am worse than before for it. I even had to have an additional second surgery for it. It is high risk operation that does not always work!" Well, the surgeon had told me that this is a complicated operation and that it has some risk. "They do not know of the outcome, and they do not always tell you everything!"

Pete had ended up on a wheelchair for a few months. He spent the next hour to go through details with me. As always, he knew what he talked about and he cared. After all, we had a lot in common.

For some twist of faith both our parents and expensive private schools had put the fear God in our hearts at the childhood about sex. The picture that they had depicted was nothing less than equating the "Sex Equals Death" warning that I had just gotten from my cardiologist.

We were told in details about all possible venereal diseases. We were brainwashed that sex should be only after marriage and that it is a lot more pleasurable then as opposed to causal and irresponsible sex. "As kids from reputable families, you men are expected to do the honorable things at all times!"

To really hit the point home, they showed us the nightmarish syphilis and other movies. Then there was a full length movie called the "Grandeur of Grass" with French subtitles since some of the class was more fluent in French than English.

This movie shows the consequences of being "sexually active" before the end of college. The consequence is that if you had sex in college, then you will not complete your studies and forever you will be doomed to a life bounded by mental and financial poverty.

Then there was a copy of Readers' Digest that said sex can become just as pleasurable as drinking a cold beer in summer if it is not in the context of love and marriage.

So, in the interest of time, I should have not given up on Roya. I should have found her. Then, I should have quickly fallen in love again since the award would have been extremely pleasurable sex forever, and ever.

"Bryce, are you still there?" on the phone brought me back to being almost sixty and having all these sensual and sexy thoughts. I resumed my conversation with Pete. He had the same attitudes about sex.

Like me, he too had really wanted to marry the day he graduated. But that too was not in the cards. His sweetheart was Megan.

All this depravation had caused both of us to go into a feeling of emptiness that we thought perfect sex with the most attractive women could heal. After all Barry White sings a song called "Sexual Healing".

Almost every TV ad shows a half naked sexy woman pitching, one product or the other. This bombardment of visual aphrodisiacs is nonstop and potent.

Somehow a transition happens and we go from sex deprived to the one that thinks about sex every five minutes; as someone who tries to undress each attractive woman we see with our eyes; or as the case with Dean Martin, try to guess how their panties look like. The urge is billions of years old and it is hardwired in our brains.

Thus we have entered the era of sex craze!

But the more sex we are lucky to get, the more emotional empty we start to feel. Thus, we need to get more as if the next sex will be that sex act that heals all our emotions regarding sex and makes us complete.

Each sex act ends with us losing interest in our one night stand lover, and thinking about the next. We plan for the next time to be up in the sky during a flight. When that does not quite satisfy, then we might try to have sex in a parking lot risking detection. When that does not quite do the trick, we plan to have sex in an elevator. I did all of these.

Unfortunately, right now, I am sentenced to sexual deprivation.

Along with the sexual revolution of the sixties, we also got an epidemic of sexual depression induced by sexual envy. Unlike before that nobody was having sex; the sexual revolution made it OK for everybody to have sex all the time. Moral and spiritual standings were pushed aside. It seemed like everybody did it.

More accurately, it seemed like everybody was doing it. As a result, decent and good men like Pete and I were left out. At least this was what we thought. Yes to family values and Expectations meant no to sex!

Many years ago, Alcoholic Anonymous, which was one of the first to understand alcoholism as a disease and offer a practical recovery plan, had also some side program like sexual addiction and sex and love addict programs.

We had just finished talking about surgery that Pete asked me how everything else was. Then he abruptly changed the subject and asked, "Do you remember Mick Jagger's song?"

"Yes, the one that says I get no satisfaction!" "I am planning a last Tango in Paris with a side trip to Amsterdam. What do think?" He had no problem connecting dots together and asked, "Amsterdam as in Red Light District?" Just so I would not appear like an idiot, I added "Of course there are plenty of tourist places to see too."

His immediate reaction was, "Why not!"

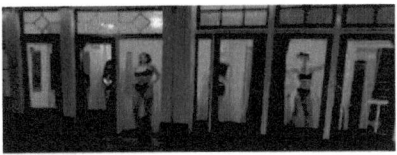 CHPATER 7: Amsterdam
Red Light District

Pete's concurrence gave me courage and permission to live my last months on this earth; not to be a living dead before I died. I had every right to want to enjoy and have fun in my last months on this earth. Actually, my last "quarters of life", meaning I had only six to nine months to live since each quarter is three months. Thinking about enjoyment of life, catapulted me into my vivid remembrance of my trip to Amsterdam Red Light District when I was twenty-seven. I had arrived in Amsterdam as horny as hell! Somehow all the pain of a broken loving relationship with Roya, had transformed it into my desire to have sex here with what looked like sexiest women on earth. These were professionals; the sex artists; the practitioners of perfect and fulfilling sex; the real life fulfillment of satisfaction that only sex could provide as seen on movie screens.

The KLM flight from Heathrow had several stunningly attractive flight attendants. Somehow, the interior design of the DC9 aircraft had pastel colors that were appealing to eyes. Not just appealing, but alluringly and sexy as well. I was so sex deprived, so love stricken with Roya, and so depressed that I could have made love to the aircraft. The inside of the plane had a sensual scent as well that intensified my sex drive. To my distorted and thirsty sex drive, the scent inside that KLM airplane seemed to be similar to the lavender mixed with Chanel Number 5 that was typical of a certain brand of lubricated condoms.

We arrived in Amsterdam Schiphol Airport at 10:00 AM on an overcast day. Most English speaking passenger pronounce Schiphol as "Skip Hole" since they cannot pronounce this the way Dutch do. Dutch has many guttural sounds including the "Kh" that is written as "ch."

I went to my hotel room and took a shower. Then, I carefully studied the maps and books. Soon, I was on my way to finally consume what billion years of evolution and Madison Avenue Advertising had subliminally brain washed me.

I was on my way to get that one and only most important experience in life of having sex with some of the most attractive women in the world. It was as serious rite of passage as anything else in the world. As a man, we had to have this passionate, urgent, and burning desire that is closest to the heavenly pleasures relieved. This made the temptation and drive overwhelmingly stronger since this pleasure, even earthly, was closest to what you could find only in heaven. I had to experience this or die. I had to become a man rather than a virgin boy!

Suddenly, I remembered hundreds of films, including the "Top dog" that men did the most heroic things risking their lives. Then they would chase, and finally find that perfectly photographed Venus and be privileged enough to make love to her.

But these Venuses did not look like this in their real lives. I knew. I had been in movies. It took a crew of people to "Create or Formulate" such beauties on the screen.

Then, I quickly realized that I was a man in heat, and I needed to consume my burning desires for sex.

By then, I found myself window shopping in Amsterdam Red Light District. The first window, I passed quickly. She was pretty all right. But she was not my type. I stopped and almost turned back to apologize to her for rejecting her. Then I realized again that this was Red Light District.

The second window, one look and it looked somebody had poured kerosene on my entire body and had lit a fire at the same time. I was burning with passion, desire, and anticipation of sex.

She showed the door to me and gestured me to enter. I hesitated. I told myself this is not ethical. "This is sin as bad as any sin can be. This is not right! No, this is not for someone like me!" Then as if to complete the argument, I told myself "Maybe I cannot even afford it!"

It seemed and felt like my legs were uncontrollably dragging the rest of my body towards her door. It did not matter what I thought, or what ideology or reasoning I was feeding myself, my body wanted pleasure, fulfillment, satisfaction, and even was taunting me that this was my chance to become a man and not stay a boy! "You are still a boy until you lose your virginity. Then, and only then you become a man!"

It was an "Out of Body" experience. It felt as if my feet were walking a few steps ahead of me. In fact, as my hand reached to open the door, it felt for a moment that my legs -with what was erect in between my legs – had already entered the room, or more precisely entered that lovely woman.

By now, my entire body, and I were in the room.

"Twenty Guilders!" she said. Then added more, depending on what else you want done! She spoke perfect English with some accent that I later learned to be Dutch. She then rushed to add "You need to pay cash, in advance, and in Dutch currency!"

This seemed like one of those Hollywood movie lapses. I had been standing and talking to her one moment, and the next moment, cut, she was unrolling a condom on my fully erected penis.

Since I was standing there like a statue, she decided that in the interest of time, she could satisfy me standing up. These sex artists, according to confession of one of the Beatles, could read your mind – no matter how dirty your mind was, read your sexual feelings, and they could speak to your body in a very sensual language. By training or experience, they have learned how to give you your heart's delight before you could ever express that in words.

As I entered her, then I gently moved forward to kiss her sexy lips. "No! No! I am sorry we have to stop! Nobody is allowed to kiss me on the lips! That is reserved for my boyfriend!" This made me surprised, disappointed, and made me feel a strong case of "coitus interruptus". Coitus interruptus is a rudimentary birth-control technique in which a man withdraws his penis from a woman before ejaculation during sex so that the seaman is not ejaculated inside the pussy. She gently pushed back enough so my penis that was fully erected would slide out of her beautiful and nicely lubricated pussy. The sensation during this short slide was extreme pleasure along with anger and apprehension for not being completely satisfied. As I was coming out of her, I lost my erection and the condom fell down. As I was trying to find an answer to why this had happened since we had an agreement for a consensual sex, she added "Only my boyfriend is allowed to do that!" She then gently touched me, and I was burning hot and boiling. A few seconds later, she gave me a kiss on my chick followed by a full-fledged and intensely passionate French kiss. "I can tell that you badly needed that kiss to warm up. Please do not tell anybody about this kiss!" Kissing or not, I felt that I was coming with what felt like hot soup gushing out of me, and splashing on some bullet proof material that the condoms were made from. Finally, I was not a virgin boy any more. Finally, I was a man. Furthermore, finally I had become a man without begging or pushing a woman.

The ejaculation lasted a lot longer than usual since that French kiss had done its magic. She took a towel and made it wet with some hot water, let it sit for a few seconds, and then she used that to clean me up. Then as I was flat on my back on her bed, she took another towel and put cold water on it and started to wrap it around my fully erect penis. She whispered something like, "honey, you are still hot. I cannot let you get out of my room with an erect penis. She put some more lipstick on her beautiful lips, and then planted a second French kiss before I could ask for it to warm me up. She had read my mind loud and clear. Then she applied some foundation powder that only looks good on her type of light Northern European complexion. This adds another ten Guilders! "No problem, please go ahead." Then she climbed on the bed and on top of me. In a fraction of a second, I was totally inside her. I felt at that moment that I had the biggest penis of any man in the world. I was a proud man about my manhood while I was inside her. She managed to sit on top of me for better penetration while she was refreshing her chocolate-bronze lipstick.

A few moments of riding me, and riding me hard, she carefully changed her position so tip of my penis would hit her clit, and then instantly, she would budge just so little that my penis would glide past her fully engorged clit. Right about then, she would make a slight movement sideways and push down so ever gently that my penis would enjoy the deepest penetration I had ever experienced in my entire life.

Somehow, I could not come and she was watching the time carefully. Her solution was simple. She got off and took the condom off my penis. She got a new condom and rolled it on my shy but fully erected penis after using the towel with cold water to wipe it off.

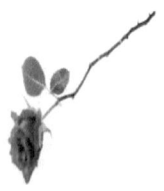

With a big smile on her face, she told me to relax. What I did not know then, but I learned a lot later was that a lot of these women carefully present their pussy, or even rub it on your face to get you excited. She sat on the edge of the bed, and gently asked me to watch her pussy in the mirror.

Just like a doctor diagnosing a complicated case, she said that I was not getting enough friction. Then she rubbed her finger on the foundation powder and rubbed it carefully and sensually on her pussy near the labia, and some right inside. Then she took a bit of time to smooth this out and applied some more lipstick on her labia and right inside.

Before I knew it, she was on top again. She was right the friction was doing its job. While this was going on her beautiful breasts, each with a thick layer of lipstick on each nipple was jumping up and down with each movement of hers. A few attempts at this, she decided this was not working. She got off, and hurriedly brought a small bottle of lubricant and removed the seal and squeezed a lot in between her shapely breast; she repeated this process on both from the top and then bottom side of her cleavage. When she was putting this lubricant on, I felt that I urgently needed to learn to do what I heard from other boys in school to be a "Tit Sex!"

Then she asked something that my sizzling, dark red, overheated ears were not capable of hearing. "Do you like me to put on my panties?" was her question that she had to repeat with the hope of getting an answer from me. I was so highly excited that my best effort generated a little noise that she could not decipher. She, at that point, seemed to be in as much heat as I was. She was indeed hot to throat. Without wasting any time, she murmured something to herself like. "OK, then, in that case, I will wear one!"

A very clean white Olga bikini style panty, with one itsy bitsy rose on the left side came out of the top drawer almost flying out. When she forced the drawer to close it, I was sure that she was hot for me too or she was one of those very few women who indeed liked sex! With condom off, my penis got over excited by watching this stunningly beautiful and sexy woman. I had my second ejaculation gushing from underneath her breasts like a fountain in about three minutes right inside her breast from the bottom. Her reaction was, "too bad, this was a bit too fast for both of us. You need to get more practice, or buy a special spray from the sex shop nearby."

Her shining strawberry blonde hair was flying in the air reflecting the indirect light like a mirror. Her Turquoise blue eyes were out of this world. What took a few minutes, seemed like a fraction of second to me.

I was done, satisfied, and finally I had become a certified man! I thought that I was the luckiest man on earth at that moment, because she was indeed one of the sexiest and prettiest women in the world.

I thanked her, and forcefully pushed myself out of her room. The room that was extremely clean and the room that had been my kingdom of coming of age!

I walked almost aimlessly for a while. I had the taste of her lipstick, and feel of her strikingly desirable and sexy lips on my mouth. After a few minutes of walking, I wanted, and desperately wanted to go back for more and more! Then I arrived at a place where tourists could ride on one of the famous Amsterdam Canal Sightseeing Boats. Bergman is one of the companies that have canal tours almost every hour. Unknown to tourists, they take pictures of tourists as they board this relatively big boat. Then they developed them, and sell them to you when you disembark. When, I saw my picture, I was convinced that I had to buy this picture. Not only to buy, but also to keep and cherish it forever. After all, this picture was proof positive that moments before I had became a man. Not only I had become a man, but I was lucky to have had sex with one of the sexiest women in the world. This was Right next to my birth certificate; this was my becoming a man evidence and indisputable certificate of manhood.

This picture was something else too. It empowered me to be strong and not to let devastating effects of Roya's loss to emotionally kill me. I was alive again. I was trying to heal my emptiness; I was trying to heal my deep and painful wounds; I was on my road to recovery.

In that canal tour, I was sitting next to a fascinating woman who was there with her husband. She was attractive. Much to my surprise, I was not paying any attention to her. I had just become a man and I was flying in cloud nine. I was not envious of the handsome man sitting right next to her who had such a pretty wife anymore.

As the brand new Bergman tourist boat was passing the Bloomen Mart, which is a flower market, I decided to buy some flowers for my most beautiful partner for that night that I became a man! Not just a man, but a world class and high class at that man! Soon I had to remind myself this was Red Light District, and the thirty Guilders was my entire obligation in that enormously pleasurable give and take.

Suddenly, as if I was hit by a rock, the growling in my stomach was a red alert reminding me of my dire hunger. I found something to eat quickly and was back to my hotel room.

Next day, and the day after that was spent in carefully selecting the most attractive women in the world and getting that instant gratification that I could only see, and therefore imagine how it might feel in Hollywood movies!

I had heroically conquered that one and only one thing that is the most important Hollywood thing in this world! I had quenched my visually induced hallucination of sexual gratification.

The fourth day, I had sex with a tall lady with curly red hair. This was a natural red hair, nothing like to those punk rockers. Her red bikini had a unique red color. As I was trying to figure out what shade it was, I was abruptly stopped in my tracts! Oh my God. Oh my God, Oh my God, this was the Fire Engine Red color that Roya was talking about. This was one and the same as the color of that Ford Mustang that I was supposed to get!

Wow! What a twist?

A moment of hesitation came and went quickly. I had returned to this woman's room for the second time. She recognized me and asked "Here for more of the same, or you like something else?" I pleaded, "No, no, the same as last time!" Unimpressed, she took the money, pushed it inside some notebook, and helped me undress.

The second act was consumed! The pleasure sensation was nothing less than taking off like a spaceship, going to the outer space of the ultimate in higher joy, and then coming down back to earth. Not only this was most erratic, and enjoyable, and satisfying, but it also made me proud of myself. I was proud of every inch of my existence. Interesting thing is that had I not been there myself, I would have considered this a large tale if I ever heard it from another person. However, every second of it was real and exciting.

After that boat ride, I went for my walk. The energy was so high in this woman that I was in sweats. I had not broken a sweat with other women. This woman was insanely full of energy and desire. She too wanted more and more of it. It seemed like she wanted it all the time. As I was being calmed down as a result of the relaxing walk, I discovered the reason. I had discovered reason and not sensational imagination portrayed by Hollywood to all those hungry eyes immersed into purely visual pleasure. There was no touching and no feeling. It was just watching something great.

Only after that invigorating walk, and only then, reason became even more and more obvious. She was intense. She was intense in everything that she did. Nevertheless, that intensity was not it all.

I realized that while we were having sex, she without even asking started to French kiss me passionately and profusely. Her kisses were really enticingly sexy. It seemed obvious to me that she was trying to reward me for being a returning client. Or, she too as a human being, just like all other human beings also had sexual needs that she wanted to fulfill. Feelings and sexual needs that she could not somehow satisfy with others even though she was having sex ten or twenty times a day.

I decided not to tell her what others had told me about kissing on the lips. For a moment I lulled myself into telling myself maybe she does not know this. Then, I told myself, "Bryce you are not that stupid to break your silence and tell her about kissing that others did not do while the most intense sexual act in my life was being played out!" I had quickly convinced myself that I should just rejoice and enjoy each and every kiss now.

At the end of the act, right after when I was begging her to stop since I had become highly sensitive after climax, I decided to tell her about inadmissibility of kisses as others had told me. Honesty was the best policy. Was it not?

I noticed that she put her clothes on and sat on her chair right near her tiny round make up table. The mirror on the wall helped me see her beautiful face as she was applying lipstick. "You took all my lipstick away! This seldom happens. Let me tell you, you are something, you are strong, and you are the caring type! Then, she had to switch to French and say that I was romantic. I was romantic, European style. Well, romantic European when told to an American by a European means is a serious complement! It must be a rare complement!

She was French. She had lived in Amsterdam for a very long time. This she told me in French. In fact she was so surprised that I, and American, spoke French. This was quite a unique one in a thousand thing that she had seen.

I almost left the door, but then I made a sudden U turn and slowly approached her. "May I?" Before she could say anything, this time I gave her a long affectionate kiss. Then, I gave her another kiss that somehow ended up being not so affectionate. "This one is to say thanks" I said.

I noticed she was shaking her head. "I told you, you are sensitive and hopelessly romantic!" Then putting her hand over mine, she whispered, "You are hopeless, but special!"

I had planned to go to the Aviodom which is an aviation museum near Schiphol Airport. As I looked at different airliners and flight attendant uniforms, I kept being reminded of the more perfect than perfect sex that I had with one of the prettiest and most gentle sexual artists in the world.

This was sexual healing as Barry White says in his songs.

My plans were to get a dinner in a nice restaurant and go to bed early next day since I wanted to go to Rotterdam which is a lovely and famous port. In the Dutch folklore, they say that "God created the entire world except Holland!" Then they add that "Dutch created Holland!" This is not a boast. Holland, which is called "Low, or Down Country" in French transliteration is several hundred feet below the sea water level. A delicate network of canals has reclaimed inch of land by inch from the cold and bitter North Sea to create the fertile Dutch soil.

Last minute, like a tiny pin that was pulled by irresistible pull of a huge magnet, I looked into several windows hoping to find my red haired sex lover!

The more I looked the less successful I was. Being dinner time, it seemed that most had gone out for dinner.

"OK Bryce, enough is enough. If you are still excited, then go find another beauty!" I told myself as if trying to calm down a crying three-year old who was crying to get candy.

I took a cab and went to have a sit down dinner at a nice restaurant in the train station. In most of European cities, the train stations are still the center of the city culture, shopping, trade, and with walking distance from just about anything.

I unconsciously found myself back in the Red Light District as if I had sleep walked myself there!

I noticed the set of windows that were sort of like the place that my red hair lover was. I had to find her. I was disparately longing and yearning for her intimate and intense love making again. I was madly obsessed and even felt deprived.

Most windows were now dark as it was late in the night. Another shift would have started later on.

Insistently, my well known psychological "Child Within" had thrown a tantrum. Like a spoiled two year old, it demanded sex and intimacy and wanted it badly wanting the Red Hair Magic! This was a rage that could only be satisfied by her.

I was noticing yet another closed window, when I heard a door opening!

I was about to walk away, as I noticed that the light came on! My goodness! It was my red haired intense lover! This was the same lover that having had sex with twice had not satisfied me yet that day.

The third time was a kind of record.

"Are you up to it? Maybe your eyes are bigger than your abilities!" I decided if I could not perform for the third time, I pay her and just ask her all those burning questions that I had about sex all these years!

Maybe being a sex artist with unlimited experience she could answer some of my puzzling questions!

Suddenly to my ultimate delight, I realized that the door that had opened behind me was her door. As if I had been beamed up from where I was standing outside and then beamed down in her room and literally in her arms, I had arrived!

She told me that she knew that I would come back for the third time! She knew this so well, that she did not go home in her usual time and she waited for me.

"Would you like me to teach you something advanced?" Wow!

Just not to hurt my fragile male ego seared with envy, she said only one percent of men know this method. You intrinsically know it, but I like to help you refine it.

"To make love to woman, you have to read her like a newspaper." "Remember, if you were there just to have sex, you will sooner or later, get tired of it!" Then whispering in my ear, she said you "must love the woman who is having sex with you if at least during the act, if not forever!"

Then another startling fact appeared in her answer to my next question.

I asked her how was I in comparison to other men. As a typical man, my question was painfully direct and stupid. What I was really asking her was "Was I long enough and thick enough compared to other men!" This of course did keep in mind that she must have seen hundreds of men of different shape and size.

Let us enjoy the third time, and I will give you answer after that.

Intensity this time was sky high. Her kisses were like lifesaving intravenous infusions. She was magically moving her body at the speed of light, but her lips were stationary and her kisses were even more passionate than before.

I had submitted my body and soul to her for complete and super gratifying surrender!

It felt as if I had not had sex for months and months even though I had sex with her just hours ago and then hours before that.

This was indeed the third time, and I had performed with flying colors.

But my male ego boosted my false pride was elevating not because of me. It was in fact in spite my inhibitions and brainwashing from primary school.

As I was trembling again with delight, and almost fainting, I learned my lesson. I am a man. I am a man no different than the others. My medieval desires for sex are natural. I cannot deny them, I cannot burry them, and I cannot live with or without them. When in college, a doctor told me that as a man we all have this biological and psychological urge. However, we also have the need to be responsible and sensible.

No use fighting.

The Red Hair gave me a hug. This hug was caring, smooth, and meant a lot to me. It helped me feel that I had not just gone to market, paid, and bought something. It felt like a human to human interaction had deeply taken place.

I wondered what if I took her back to the US with me. I had heard that this is one of the greatest most rewarding acts of kindness rewarded in several religions.

At this peak of delight, pleasure, sexual healing or fulfillment, she gave me another touching hug and another passionate kiss!

"Before I forget, I owe you an answer."

She was referring to my stupid question regarding my manhood being as long, or as thick, in Inches or in Centimeters as she was French and they used metric system. At this point I felt like mine was the biggest and the best and no other man were any bigger or better.

She said the "Honest answer is that…" A long pause to make sure she has my hundred or more percent attention followed. "Every man is different!" Then with big emphasis, she said "Each and every man that she or another woman in that district had had sex with, are and always remain the longest and thickest since each man is different!"

This was indeed out of this world. She said and meant it too, "Every man is different!"

She meant different in good way and not bad.

Years later something else clicked with me. Some women feel like virgins no matter how much sex they have had. This is a miracle of the nature. Their vagina almost always remains and is as elastic and supple as when they were very young virgins. This miracle of nature has been medically established.

I am positive that my Red Hair Sensational Typhoon must have been one of those. In fact that was one of the things that she told me, but I did not take that serious.

Having sex with her was something surreal!

As part of my therapy, I had talked about my experience with my trusted therapist. Of course, the conversation would always be clean, polite, and clinically cold. Most of the time, she would try to put things in perspective for me. At times she would say that the sex drive is the most beautiful thing that we as human beings have. She would then add that feelings related to sex and relationships are highly complicated. Like Pete, she too never judged and never took sides. However, talking about some of my most deep sexual secrets seemed to immensely help me free myself from the associated pain and shame.

There is a saying that you will get tired of sex after a while. This reality manifested itself later on during my day eight in Red Light District saturated sex odyssey.

On the eighth day, it was the trip to Rotterdam. During my trip to Rotterdam, I had noticed there was a house - an ordinary house - that had an open window. That window opened to some woman's bedroom. Looking a bit closer, I noticed a super attractive woman sitting right in the window. The surprising thing was that as some men were passing by, some just stopped and talked to her briefly. But most of them just walked on. One, in fact walked away as if he had heard something insulting from the beautiful woman. He was a shorter man with a colorful tie wearing and an old faded jacket walking with a limp. He had not shaved for a few days, and he had forgotten to comb his unruly hair.

Curiosity was getting to me. I had to inspect this a bit further. This was a younger woman in a nice satin night gown. She had a fresh makeup and her hair was just perfect.

The fact was that after having had sex with my red haired sensation, it sort of felt like I had had enough for a while. The trip to Rotterdam was supposed to be a touristy act by me. Rotterdam is a world-class port and it is really worth seeing. So, it was sort of reasonable to give sex a rest, at least for one day.

I also quickly remembered that the day before I had had sex with this ultra sexy red hair woman, I had one of those least satisfying ones with a very tall and cold blonde. She seemed to not have any expression on her face, and no warmth on her body. I was feeling particularly responsible. I was busy damning myself. My money was responsible to bring this woman here. Who knows, she could be one of those trafficked women who was deceived and brought here by evil men. Sex with her was joyless, purely mechanical, and even discouraging. The only word exchanged after the rate was set, was her question at the end. Her question was, "Did you just come?"

Therefore, by then I should have theoretically had enough "Window Shopping" that should have lasted weeks, months or even years. To some extent it had lost its glamour, and I was delightfully tired. So, the day trip to Rotterdam was to be a respite from saturated sex.

Nevertheless, I did not know what to do when it came to this movie star looking woman a few feet from me. I was a bit tired. The physical act of sex does demand high activity from almost all the mussels in our bodies, including the ones in my head!

She had noticed that I had been carefully watching her from a distance. Therefore, she was somewhat more approachable to me than the others as if I was more important or serious.

As I got closer to the window, I realized that she had no bra under that purely white satin night gown. The room also had a very fresh lavender scent. This scent was not too overpowering, and it was not too faint either.

The bedspread was also made of a tasteful nude color satin matching the pillows on this queen sized bed.

There was a nice and organized book shelf with mostly Dutch books. But soon I detected the famous American book "The Joys of Sex" on the top shelf.

As I slowly and carefully walked towards her, she applied another layer of fresh lipstick to her sexy and highly desirable lips.

As I was a few feet away, I heard she ask "Do want to put your lipstick into my hot lipstick cover?" This turned me on unbelievably. I was as hard as I ever was and instantly!

Feeling like a miner who has suddenly discovered the biggest diamond mines on earth, I just froze.

I would give an arm and a leg to go to bed with this woman. But, this unlike Red Light District was a private house. There was no sign outside. What is more the small garden right outside was immaculately kept.

What is going on?

I was feeling unprepared and suspecting a scam. Then I faintly remember that in one of those tour books there was sentence about private sex parlors in Amsterdam and other Dutch cities.

She had gladly detected that I was not as innocent as I had originally appeared walking towards her window and that I might be serious enough. She added, "I normally charge 200 Guilders for one hour. One hour of whatever your little heart desires, except for hurting me or you. S&M, I mean serious S&M – again without hurting – can cost as much as 400 for that hour. But, today, I will you the hour for 150 instead of 200! Come on in you will be happy!"

First things first, as always, business has to be first. I carefully counted and placed the 150 Guilders in a small nice silver plated plate.

She then called a name. This was a Dutch name, but to my surprise and angst, it was a man's name. I knew enough to realize this from the name alone.

A very clean-shaven gentleman entered the room after knocking three times in rhythm.

She, in passing introduced him to me as her husband!

Her husband!

What? How could this be? How this could be her husband showing up right before the sex act was to begin? Right before my lipstick could go into her cool, soft, and most satisfying lipstick cover?

Seconds later he bent and gave his wife a semi-passionate kiss. His kiss was nowhere as passionate as the ones I had gotten from my red hair, permanent virgin sex lover. His were much more like a caring husband kissing his wife before going on a business trip. There was enough passion to say I love you, but too much to entice the wife into sexual desire for sex right there and then. It was more like I love you but I have to go.

I lost my erection.

As a person who had lived in dangerous parts of New York City, I intuitively knew that I had to retreat. "Leave the money and escape with your life!"

Then starting to tell myself that it has been a nice life to prepare myself for death or complete disfigurement, I noticed that the husband was politely extending his hand to me for a handshake.

"Shake his hand! Shake his hand! Cooperate! This must be a professional killer. Do not do anything that would aggravate him!" Hurry up, shake his hand! Smile if you have to, it could save your life. Do it. Do it now! Now, now, do not hesitate it could cost your life!"

Even though I was heroically extending my best effort, I could not fool the husband or the wife!

"Mr. Condon, your life is about to end! This time sex could be fatal! You had this coming!"

The husband, as if he had woken up from sleep during an earthquake of magnitude 8.5, backed off and said something alarming to his wife on the bed.

"Excuse me sir. You are here because of our ad in the adult newspaper?" He was begging to know. My terse reply to his bewildered question was "What ad?"

A rapid fire of Dutch/Flemish went back and forth.

I noticed they both looked at me with sympathy. More precisely, they were more horrified than I was.

The man reached for the small silver plate. He slowly lifted it and very slowly walked towards me. The woman got off the bed and gave me a very passionate kiss.

I was going crazy. What was happening!

The woman, who seemed to better educated, explained slowly. She said that she was married to this man. Yes he is my husband and I love him dearly. Then she added that they routinely placed ads in the adult newspapers for sex. Then she added that I was perhaps familiar with having sex with just one woman. But a more intense form of sex is between multiple partners. Some men have sex with two women at the same time.

I politely said, "I understand" as if my life depended on it. I had more reason to fear losing my dear life as the window was shut and the curtain was closed.

The man in a very caring way told me, "We thought that you were here for a threesome."

What he meant was that I would have direct or indirect sex with the husband as well as direct sex with the wife.

The money in the plate was slowly moving towards me as if in slow motion in movies or sports events as my brain had gone into high gear to just figure out what was happening.

The woman had now moved right near me touching my hair and giving me a sensual hug right in front of his husband. Again my gaze fell on her beautiful shapely nude breasts. I had sensed with all my physical and emotional being that her silky skin must feel just like fresh cream. The coloration of her skin and hair reminded me of Angelina. I noticed the way her slippery night gown was gliding over that ultimate soft skin. By that time her night gown had opened up, and I could see that she was totally nude under it.

I was dying to touch her, even if her husband would kill me. Then the thought was what if he also wanted to have direct sex with me. Whatever direct or indirect meant in that context! The answer hit me, and hit me hard right away. I was not interested in direct sex with another man.

They were apologizing.

The husband said that he thought the best would be for me to have one hour party with his wife. Shook my hand and left the room. Then he quickly came back and said he felt so bad about their mistake that he would return all the money and I will have the one hour party with his wife for free.

By then, I was convinced that they were sincere. I started to feel sorry for them. However, I was feeling totally safe with them at that point.

I had an exciting memorable, intimate, seductive sex hour is another man's bed, and with another man's wife! It was all three way consensual, safe, and even semi-ethical yet classy.

"What, repeat that last sentence, again! You are telling me you had sex with a man's wife in his bed and while he was sitting drinking beer in the next room? And, you are alive to talk about it?" These were Pete's reaction upon my return. At that instant, it seemed like I had outdid the sexual and romance champion of the century.

To continue with the story, I must add the husband invited both of us to a cold bear afterwards.

Few minutes after the beer was finished, she invited me to a shower with her. After taking a quick shower with me, they were now in the bed together and begging me to stay. But they clearly told me that I did not have to participate it I did not wanted.

I chose not to participate. But that cite seeing exercise trumped all other cite seeing tours I have ever had anywhere in the entire world in my entire life.

They were like artists. Well, they were really artists, sex and romance artists. They were choreographed to anticipate and engage magnificently in each and every minor or major movement of each other in bed. She was experiencing multiple real orgasms. They were not faking it. Sometimes they were coming together.

I had seen "Live Sex Acts" back home in the movies and really live in Amsterdam before, but nothing like this megawatt energy act in bed room live and close cite seeing. I had always thought how sexy it could be if I could somehow see what married couples or just plain sexual partners did in the privacy of their bedroom. This was one in a million chances to see it up close! My watching them do their act was turning them on with a fiery passionate sex. During the act, the bed would shake as if there had been an earthquake. Yet these shakes felt as soft and creamy as a sexy woman's skin.

They seem to notice the slightest body or eye movement on my part and they would move or act somewhat differently as if to give me a better view to try to reignite my desires and join them after all.

I must admit that temptation was intense and burning. However, I already had more than my fill. I was fully satisfied. Because of that, I did not have any sexual anxiety while I was enjoying watching their superb lover's act.

I decided to accept their invitation to take a shower. Then she offered something else. "Considering heavy sex that you have had, I strongly recommend that you apply this on. This keeps you cool and prevents you from burning later on." She took a towel and gingerly tapped it on my semi-erect manhood to dry it. Then she applied what just looked like a lipstick to cover it entirely. Talcum powder was applied just enough where it was most appreciated and then there was a final touch.

She took a pancake out of her foundation powder container and applied just a bit on each side. Just enough powder so I will have a taste of sensuality. Then it was time for me to put my brief on. Before I could zip my pants, she took one of her panties which had a slight lavender scent, and gently folded it so the crutch would be inward and in touch with me at all times.

Bull Durum was a movie that had a part just like this. This fictional basketball player could only win if he had this type of panties touching him.

The red lipstick had had a cooling sensation on me. But each move and each time her panties came in touch with me, it felt exactly, precisely like that moment that my lipstick was softly gliding into her lipstick cover. This was imaginative, virtual, and artificial sex! Thinking back, TJ from Sheri's Ranch had told me that imagination is the bigger part of having sex.

I kept her panties for many, many years.

Incidentally, I have never talked to my therapist about this encounter. I do not know why to this day. Furthermore, I must say that after this, I was hundred percent satisfied. The sensational arousal and the touching sensation were so strong that I had never been able to duplicate them ever.

One of the Beatles was talking about the great satisfaction he had from having sex with "Sexual artists." In this instance, I seem to have done much better than the Beatles. Not only I had been in bed and had sex with a sexual artist, I had a finely performed acrobatics, ballet dance, and artistic romantic sex of the most satisfying kind.

That extended fireworks is still alive in my one-track mind as well as my soul.

Each of her refined movements, motions, or just simple moans did something to sky rocket fire the sexual sensation experience.

Upon my return to Hotel Temmel in Amsterdam, I thought that I had enough for at least some time and I should go back home to save some money.

There is a big KLM office right next to the Bloomen Mart, in one of the main streets in Amsterdam. I went in to see if I could fly back earlier.

I was not completely sure. As I was standing in line, I realized that there were many other cite seeing that I had not done yet.

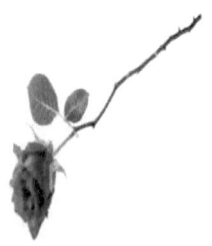

Finally, it was my turn to talk to the agent. I immediately noticed her beautiful cleavage. I also noticed that she had a type of lipstick color that I had never seen before. It was a combination of chocolate, lavender, purple, and light and dark brown that made it extremely unique. Her purple dress accentuated her beautiful greenish blue eyes.

Voices in my brain went into hyperactivity. "You might think you have had enough, but you did not!" Then, to prove the point, they shouted, "Go home and you will forever and ever be sorry." After that came the warning, "No one ever gets enough of this!"

After the KLM agent had taken a look at the ticket and checked something in her computer, she started to talk to me. She said, "There is enough space in daily flight for you tonight which leaves in six hours." "Unfortunately, because you had a super-saver ticket, there will be a 300 Guilder penalty. I can do this for you now if you like."

Before I would hear voices shouting in my ears again, I told her that I had decided not to change. I will stay. While 300 Guilders might sound a great deal, nevertheless, I could not extinguish the desire filled thought that I could have 15 sex parties instead with 15 different gorgeous and sexy women in the Red Light District.

The intensity of the Rotterdam treatment was so high, that I decided not to go to the Red Light District the next day. I decided to give it a rest. I was having split personality. Being oversexed for someone right after sexual depravation is extremely difficult. It is like torture, but it is pleasurable torture. I guess, but I do not really know.

A day trip to Alkmaar, and its world famous cheese market was fascinating.

I felt like I had overdosed on sex. During the cheese market show and cite seeing tour, I was fixated in whether I should have sex that day or not. Part of me said enough is enough. The other part said, "You did not have a vacation in many years and are suffering from the dejection caused by break up with Roya, then live a little!" Not to mention that I only had a few quarters left to live.

The bus tour stopped near a big church on the way back. This stop was heaven sent. I had promised to go back to church and beg for forgiveness for having had sex with a married man since it was against my ethical and strict upbringing. This was the chance. After having said my most sincere prayers for forgiveness, I shed some tears. These tears seemed to be tears of joy mixed with tears of sorrow. Nevertheless, I felt that a big burden was lifted from my shoulders.

That night I could not go to sleep.

At around 12:30 AM I decided to go to the Hotel Lobby just to see some other human beings to detract me from sex, sex, and more sex. I was going sex crazy! Again, I was feeling like a drug addict suffering from withdrawal anxiety combined with depression and remorse. Yet the urge to get the next fix, at any price, was overwhelmingly ruling my life at that moment.

I had become friends with the Hotel Lobby agents. I had helped one prepare for his English test needed for certification. To another one, I had given some American cigarettes.

As I was talking to them a couple entered the lobby hand in hand. The woman was seductive, sexy, pretty and very presentable. The man was old enough to be her father and somewhat unkempt but clean.

After greeting the desk agent, who had become friends with me, he got his room key and went upstairs.

After they went upstairs, the desk agent sat in another chair opposite me in the lobby. "It has been a long day, he said." I thought it was an opportune moment to ask about the couple that just went upstairs. I said, "Honeymooners?" He quickly replied "No!"

Since the woman was strikingly attractive and sexy, I was dying with envy. How man like that could take her to her room? "What did that man have that I did not?" I was dying to find out.

The desk agent started to smoke another of the cigarettes that I had given to him before. By the time he got to the middle of the cigarette he said in passing. "She is from Spain. This is her second summer in Amsterdam. She makes good money. We watch out for her. Her specialty is sixty-nine."

Oops, now it clicked. She is a sex worker! She must be. Jealousy, envy, and lust mounted a serious attack on my senses. Pretending to be cool, I asked my friend, "How much does she charge per hour?"

The answer as it was an obvious question was easy for my friend. "This is the second night that she is going to this guy's room. You might have noticed that the guy had not shaved. It is because they were going at it all night." Then to clarify, "But tonight is only one hour." I jumped in, "And how much is it per hour?" "The rate is about 200 Guilders. But, you need to negotiate. With these Spaniards, you must negotiate hard! Are you interested in having a session in your room with her?" Although this might come as a stereotype, Latin lovers are a lot more passionate. Kat from Sheri's Ranch, for example refers to Spanish as the language of love.

I heard one person coming down the stairs. It was the Spanish woman. The agent got her attention and they talked for a few minutes. Then the agent came to me and said she has another appointment but she can be here in half an hour. Can you wait?

Before I knew it, she and I were going up the steps hand in hand. My envy about the man who had been with before I did had totally dissolved in a sense of accomplishment. I was walking up the stairs with a Latino sex goddess. Her name was Rosa, which she pronounced "Rossa!"

The springs in the bed in my room were not the best made and they made lot of noise. I called it quits with her in forty-five minutes. She had previously collected the entire money for an hour and she was happy to leave even earlier.

Next day, the hotel desk clerk was sitting guests for breakfast on the relatively small dining room. Since, I was alone, and there was another man that was alone, we were assigned to the same table by him.

The man was actually Dutch. He lived in another city close to Amsterdam. He told me that he was an "Adult Business Owner." I asked "Red Light District?" He responded "yes!" Our orders for different dishes of great Dutch breakfast were ready. Half way through his breakfast, he told me that he had two girls working for him. One is upstairs and the other downstairs. The one upstairs has many repeat customers even though she charges more. On the other hand the one downstairs is more skillful.

This man afforded me a great opportunity to learn more about Red Light District. This man looked just like any other businessman. He spoke and acted just like a businessman even though his business had to do with the Red Light District sex workers.

"One of my girls decided to work for me after a terrible divorce. Her husband had beaten her regularly and forced her into rough sex. She was introduced to me by a mutual friend in our small town of Slotermeer which is about one hour away from center of Amsterdam. I gave her a loan to get an attorney for divorce. I also helped her get proper medical treatment before she started to work for me." Then he fast forwarded to today. "She has worked for me for three years now, and she is serious about a man that she met in her college. They might get married. They are really in love." He then showed me a picture of her. She was stunningly pretty. Then, as a matter of fact he added, "She has had several regulars who visit her once a month or once a week for several months now." He noticed my surprise combined with a low dose of disbelief. He looked me in the eyes and as sincerely as he could, he said "Swear to God, this is the truth. Ask the desk clerk if you do not believe me."

It clicked. He is not a pimp. He would give a room to each girl and they pay a percentage of their wages to him in return for the room and other things. He pays for clothes, cosmetics, food, regular Dr. Checkups mandated by Dutch law and other things. He told me the one upstairs has a husband and two kids. Then he added that "their marriage is as strong as a rock in spite the sex business. To them this is a business just like any other!" Then in a matter of fact he added, "These girls join me and my wife for dinner once a month. They are like my extended family. They care for me and the business and I care for them."

Regrettably, soon there came the day that I was going back home. I was happy, sexually satisfied, relaxed, and somehow proud. It felt as if I had conquered the entire world.

JFK Airport has a tiny church inside. I went there and prayed for forgiveness. Actually I prayed for more. I prayed that I had not picked up any VD on this trip.

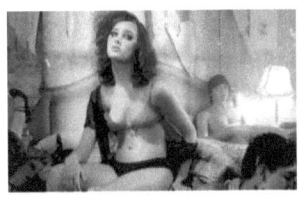

CHAPTER 8: Twelve Days of Sex Heaven

I was daydreaming about Roya.

I was trying to reconstruct events. I was struggling with the fact that it was not supposed to be. I had tried to medicate myself and all my senses into remission. This valiant trip to Europe should have healed my emotional wounds. My plans had been that as the final curtain was coming at the end of my quarters, I can tell myself "It was a nice life and now it was time to go and to go without any sexual deprivations and remorse."
Did it?
Practical facts remain that it did something. There was some magic; there was some sparkle; there was physical and emotional pleasures that exceeded any I had ever known in my life; I was a man; I was a worldly man, but something was still there unfulfilled.
It was the emptiness that could not be fulfilled with a marathon of sex with the most beautiful women in the world, not even considering that extremely unique live show in the couple's bed room. Now, the emptiness and isolation started to manifest themselves in my thoughts, imagination, and even my soul.
I had asked for and got a window seat in the DC 8 Jet. The flight officially originated in Amsterdam, and it was supposed to have New York's JFK as its final destination. However, in the sixties almost all transatlantic flights would land in Ireland's Shannon airport to refuel prior to that long flight over Atlantic.

As I was looking outside the window, I saw my image reflected in the dark night outside. It seemed to me there were three pictures of my face looking back at me. I soon figured out that most airline windows had layers of this plastic window "Glass." These three layers of glass had created reflections. This clearly explained why three pictures.

Then the thought occurred that I should be ashamed of myself. But, I had not done anything illegal. I had flown three thousand miles to go where these things were legal. Unfortunately these facts did not squelch the sadistic thought that I should be stoned. Maybe not stoned to death, but nevertheless stoned for the crime of adultery.

The thought soon expanded into the first layer. That one of those window three reflections was me. This was the "me" that deserved to be stoned. The other reflection was the "me" that was supposed to be executed by stoning. The third and last reflection, was the "me" that was asking the stoning to be done by those who had themselves not sinned!

It was like a game of Chess where three kings were in a standstill. This was standstill that was a deep and expanding quagmire.

Somehow and for reasons unknown to me the KLM flight attendant asked me if I was OK. I nodded my head trying to tell her that I was OK, when I really did not feel or believe it. An avalanche of feelings and emotions had just hit me hard. She sat right next to me and in a quiet voice asked if I was suffering from "Fear of Flying" or I was afraid of heights, or I was having a chest pain, or felt overwhelmed by anxiety. Then she told me that she only needed to know if there was an acute chest pain where they would even divert the flight to the nearest airport.

"No Madam, my heart is OK.

"Would you like me to bring you some sleeping pill, or has your Doctor ever prescribed sedative for you?

"No Madam."

She took a deep breath and then relaxed for a few seconds before going to the second stage of her questions. "Would you like to get off this flight in Shannon?" Then, she said that she thinks there is a doctor on board and if he says OK, she can get me a sedative. It is a fact that due to high population density, Dutch people have had to learn to be tolerant of each other. Also, being one of the premiere trading powers of the globe for many years, they have learned to be extremely hospitable to everyone. I could clearly sense this on this Royal Dutch Airline, KLM. KLM is a world class airline with a long history of being one of the best. This flight was no exception.

"No! Thanks for asking. I can see that this is a super world-class airline. I am OK."

She then slowly started to get up from the next seat. Half way up, she changed her mind. She sat back down and asked me if it was OK for her to keep my company. Then she explained that passenger crew ratio was such that she really did not need to serve this flight. Nonetheless, since the airline in trying to be nice, had given her the choice.

Another flight attendant appeared and asked for drinks.

I got my drink right away. The flight attendant sitting right next to me, the one that was really trying to help me could not have a drink. It was against airline policies.

"Would you like me to change your ticket so you can stay, at KLM expense, in Shannon over night? You can get a good night's rest and then you can catch the next day's flight to JFK." Before I could ask, she added that she thinks this can be done, and done easily at no charge to me. Just to assure me, she said there is a fantastic airport hotel that does a lot of business with KLM.

My first thought after the marathon sex in Amsterdam was to ask her, "Will you stay with me? We can have a lot of fun! I had just been indoctrinated with the best techniques in love making. I have the power to make you feel good!"

Half joking she added, "No, she was not included in the room deal!"

Most senior flight attendants have seen and done it all. So it was not surprising that she knew what my next question would have been. I then reached and gave her a big handshake saying this is a deal.

When we arrived, there was a KLM ground crew member with a Walkie talkie. She directed me to a waiting golf car and we were on our way to boarding an official KLM minibus that took me to the hotel.

Unlike the night before, I slept well and caught the next KLM flight. The intensity of marathon sex had finally tired me to the point that I did not have any energy left.

Finally, about an hour before landing in JFK Airport, I had the verdict. This was a judgment done by me, on myself, and the jury that was also I.

"Verdict is…" "Verdict is, not guilty of charges for the reason of being a human." That verdict indeed resolved the storm of internal conflict.

It seemed to me that bodily pleasures, regardless of commercialization of sex as a selling power, were simple and universal. What felt pleasure to an American, was more or less the same for Asian, Europeans and the others.

If we put the stigma of shame and blame aside, I had achieved a remarkable milestone in my life. A milestone that I thought might help others.

As these thoughts were occupying my mind, I decided that I acted like an ungrateful brat.

To combat this ungratefulness, I started to compose a gratitude list about the sexual pleasures received in those twelve days.

There is an American saying that says, "You cannot go back!" So, maybe, just maybe, trying to do what I could do at twenty-three may not be possible to do at fifty-eight. I had the heart problems and back pains to consider.

A few days after all these, I went to get some cash from a vending machine. I found my balance was $5,600 more than I had expected. It was my best friend Pete who must have done this.

"Pete did you put money in my account?" After a long hesitation, the answer was "Yes." He had been confined to wheelchair. As such, he did not do too much anymore. Therefore, it looked a good idea to send me a gift; his gift to for my last sexual escapade splurge. After all, his family had done great this last year.

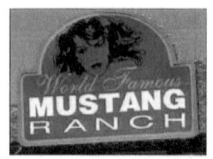 CHAPTER 9: Mustang Ranch

I was will always have found memories of those twelve intriguing, alluring, and super arousal days in Amsterdam. At the beginning, it was an experiment in finding myself, and my sexual desires. At first, I was doing what Madison Ave. subliminal and overt advertising had brain washed me to; find the blonde blue-eyed sexy, perfect woman; have perfect sex because that is the most important and satisfying reward!; go get the girl; get the girl that is not real except for in centerfold of magazines or is tampered with Photoshop, lighting, and airbrush.

Since I had never found a next door girl that matched these qualifications, I was dying to find out how sex with these painted ladies felt. Not finding these blondes that were depicted that were depicted as the essence of life for joy I was having serious depressions or blues.

According to many men, a beautiful woman may not be a sexy woman. In fact, many are convinced that Swedish blonde beauties are just as cold as ice! This is in sharp contrast to the way they are portrayed in movies such as "Swedish Fly Girls." Therefore, it just looked logical and reasonable for me to find an outlet were these elixirs for ultimate joy were. Also, most importantly as a meticulous law abiding citizen of a life time, I was not going to break the law. If the law said it was illegal, it was out of question for me. This type of puritan thinking had created a long history of depravation, anger, and frustration.

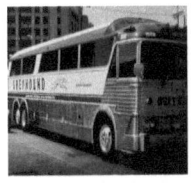 This frustration manifested itself in a sardonic and comic form as I was moving to California for the first time. Of course, as a student I did not have much money to spend. On my way to a job in California from Denver, I had high hopes of stopping at Mustang Ranch. My Greyhound bus stopped in Reno. Thus, there was perfect chance to get my fill of sexual pleasures in a clean and legal place.

This was a world famous legal bordello near Reno. I had read newspaper articles and even a new report on it. The woman did for the most part look like what I had seen in magazines. It did however shut down some years later.

I had also assumed that the Mustang Ranch might be one short taxi cab ride from the bus station. This and many other of my assumptions ended up being wrong.

Mustang Ranch was far enough from the bus station that you needed an extensive taxi cab ride. Also, there was the problem of calling a cab to pick you up after you had had your pleasure. I think that there was even a newspaper article that said a taxi cab waited with the meter running for the one hour that this "John" was having sex inside. The cab ride must have cost a great deal.

None of these made any difference. I was tired, but hot. I was going to have sex in Mustang Ranch and boast about this highest of accomplishments for the rest of my life. About an hour before we reached Reno, during one of those rest stops, I bought a Johnny Walker Red whisky bottle. It was the pocket size. In addition just not to be accused of public drunkenness, I also bought a big pack of double mint chewing gum.

Since I was sitting towards the back of the bus, I would carefully take the bottle from my jacket pocket and have a gulp in preparation for being ready when I got to the Mustang Ranch.

As I fell asleep I have a dream of Roya. Roya was out there in that Fifth Ave. boutique asking me how I brought myself to go to Mustang Ranch. Is the sexual desire so important for you to crush our ideals? Then, after a long silence, she suddenly jumped up and said, "Oh, I know what you are doing! It is a misunderstanding. I told you Ford Mustang, not Mustang Ranch. Bryce, did you ever hear of fire and brim stone? Such thing does exist. Be careful. Bryce, you are not the type. It is not worth."

I felt something press against the side of my head. That was the cold vertical bus window edge on the left that had woke me up.

Sadness sat in. I was trying to band aid a deep wound. The wound of feeling less than others who seem to have sex with those painted ladies when I could not. The wound of being told to long for sex with these beauties and to be burned each time I tried.

I had enough of this.

I did get off in Reno. Then, I decided to take a walk to think a little more. Then, to sooth my nerves, I got the pocket bottle of Johnny Walker to drink another sip. To my outrage there was nothing left. I disposed of the bottle in the first garbage container I found.

My eyes detected a cab. I almost run toward it. The driver was half sleep but happy to see me. I asked, "Sir how much to Mustang Ranch?" He looked straight into my eyes and said about $55, but we have to go with what the meter reads. After seeing the hesitation on my side, he asked "Are you going?" That was the point that I decided to trust this stranger and ask him a question. "Do you know the going rate in Mustang Ranch?" His response was like a recording, "It depends on the woman and what you want from her!" Then to qualify things so there is no doubt he added, "I have never been there myself, so I do not know." He felt sorry for leaving me in the dark like that. He then grudgingly added, "If I was supposed to guess, it is somewhere from $50 for almost nothing, to $200 to $1,000 and more." He noticed there was another passenger getting out of the bus stop. So, as he was keeping his eye on the new potential customer, he added, "I think everything included, for a nice hour of sex, with a nice 'looker woman' and the cab fare round trip, we are talking about $400 to $500, give or take $100.

"OK, thanks, let me think about this!" The driver said "No problem" but when he noticed the other passenger was getting ready to get a cab. He said OK, another cab will be here soon. May I go take these others? He was gone as soon as I said of course.

"Look at yourself! You look like a wino with that bottle." Also, to use the services of a prostitute, you have to be ashamed of yourself Mr. Bryce Condon! What if you caught something from these women? What if somebody you knew recognized you there? "

Right before going to Las Vegas, I called the bus station in Reno. "Sorry to bother you. You used to have a station manager some years ago. He was very nice to me. I wonder if I can talk to him!" I asked in a polite voice. The woman who had answered said, "It is impossible to talk to him right at this moment. But call me back in fifteen minutes after this San Francisco bus leaves, and I will try to help you. But, mister, I am not sure that I can. Call back in fifteen, will you?"

I could not wait to call back. I did and she picked up the phone right away. After reintroducing myself, she asked me exactly why I needed to contact the old station manager. "Well, you see, I had an important conversation with him many years ago. He gave me fatherly advice that has helped me a great deal all these years! I just want to say thanks." There was a quiet outburst of joy that I could not hear, but I could sense. A long pause pushed me to say "Are you still there!" A strong reaffirming "Oh, yes dear, I am here and I am just elated to hear this. The old man you are looking for is eighty-three years old now and he lives in Phoenix Arizona now. He is my dad, and I love him to pieces!" Then as if tears were coming down her face causing her voice to turn into a sad whisper suddenly, she added, "But he is not completely coherent now!"

Phoenix being the hub of the regional carriers is one of the many airports that I know like the palm of my hand. I have had to change planes there many times during my business trips.

I called and without hesitation the old man and his wife decided to meet with me. We met in a bakery and sandwich shop right there in the main concourse.

He did not seem to be that incoherent to me. We started to talk about the good old days when travel meant something. We talked about when the airline travel was a pleasurable experience. We talked about Pan American Airways and its most beautiful flight attendants. He told us about his cross country bus trip in 1948 that took about six days allowing him to do some of the best sightseeing. In fact it was that trip that made him fall in love with Greyhound and work for them forever. His wife would at times chime in to either correct something, or try to make sense of something confusing that he had said.

Among many subjects, Mustang Ranch had to come up. For this subject, he seemed to have excellent memory and seemed like his energy level went up.

"Yeah, I went there several times. There was a Tania who knew how to turn me on, keep me on, and then shoot me to the moon and back! How she did it, I do not know. I was one of her steady clients. There was another one too. I cannot remember her name. She was excellent too, but she was no Tania."

His wife could not take this anymore. She in rhetoric way asked, "Was it Tania who gave both of us the crabs shortly after we were married?" "I take the fifth on that!" was a short answer from him.

Over coffee after dinner, we talked about life. They both seemed to be proud of the fact that they were helping their daughter, the one who is now a station manager in Reno. They would tell many stories about the joys, and the heartaches involved. Then there was something unexpected that was offered.

"We had and continued to accept a less than perfect marriage. We broke up several times. We had had it with marriage and life for that matter and left each other several times. But there was some deep satisfaction that marriage, commitment, and children and only children could offer, that kept us going. I had an affair with a business owner that nearly destroyed my marriage. Once the flame and joy of doing and getting the impossible went by, she dumped me like hell. My wife was an angle to take me back."

"This is life. You cannot be logical about it. It is tough, you win and then you lose. Something works and then breaks. What you think gives satisfaction does at first and then dies. You do not always see things the way you should right there and right then. Things change. People change. Everything changes."

"Then at my age, you tell yourself that you should have tested a few of your boundaries to see if they were real or not. Life is a bitch and then we die!"

I gave each of them a hug and run to catch my flight.

As the flight took off from Phoenix Airport that night, I was remembering more and more. I remembered how on my first trip to California, I decided to retrench back to the bus station in Reno. Also how it was my luck that the station manager was not busy. In fact he seemed bored. This is the same man who just had dinner with me after all these years.

Then as I started my conversation with him, I noticed that he had a wedding ring. We started talking about the bus ride from Denver, and then seemed like quickly I changed the subject to the Mustang Ranch. Not that I wanted him to know that I was dying to go there. But, I pretended that I was just compiling general information.

He quietly told me that he had been married for a long time. Then he added that many people get off the bus, rent a car, and go there. The cab ride is too expensive. As he was talking to me, he would keep his voice as if not to let other passengers overhear what he was talking about.

Then as if he had sensed the urgency in my tone of voice, he said that it is a nice experience from what he hears. He then proudly added that he has never heard a complaint.

My attention went to his wedding ring again. It was a plain simple ring. He seemed to wear that with pride. Somehow he noticed that I was carefully studying his ring. He then added, "I do not want to appear as preaching or anything. I am not even that religious, but one thing I know for a fact. Having a loving home and kids is what it is at. The rest soon fade away." He excused himself to go and update the bulletin board.

That left me standing there wondering. As a law obedient guy who had lived with dignity, was it appropriate for me to go to a brothel? Even though this brothel was legal, I did not feel comfortable. I felt a deep agony, shame, conflicted, and remorsefully confused.

The scratchy speaker in the bus stop was announcing the departure of the next bus to Elko and points west in fifteen minutes.

Elko, on the border of California and Nevada on the Interstate 80, mean "White Girl" in Shoshone American Indian language, among other definitions.

In one radio show, talking about sexy and attractive woman, the speaker used the word "White-cy" as describing his maddening desire for a white, blonde, and blue-eyed woman. This adds fuel to the fire of men being extremely lured by blonde blue eyed women.

And then there is Hitler who had the idea that whites were the super race. Racist, sexist, and criminally sickening!

But billions of years of evolution, and sick mental programming had gotten to where I was just going crazy about having the ultimate enjoyment of life, with that perfect woman as defined by Hitler! Manikins in store windows had poured fuel to the fire everyday!

Playboy and others had also adhered to this hidden conscious or unconscious agenda. The result was that, I as an intelligent man had women, women, and women on my mind. I wanted to be loved and love that perfect Playboy centerfold. After all, men are wired to think about sex once every five minutes.

It also stood to this crooked logic that having been intimate and having made love to this goddess of perfection, everything will turn into perfect enjoyment and happy ever after. In fact, it seemed that the key to "Happy Ever After" was in the hands of these glamorous inventions, these fixations of imagination, these merchants of the "Sex Sells" school. This translated into stinky thinking that sex with an everyday real woman was indeed inferior to having sex with that blonde blue eyed elixir portrayed in TV and print. Only the blonde blue combination would satisfy the urge. This was as if this blonde blue potion will heal and satisfy men's thirst for sexual satisfaction and nothing else will do. God knows how many blonde women with blues are trafficked each year and how many of them suffer from sexual assault. I know one who told me that being pretty attracted wrong men around her all her life.

Paradoxically, when a high school student in our school was caught being memorized by these pictures of painted ladies the school expelled him for three days. This is a clear case of mixed message convoluted with double standard.

"Who knows, maybe I go there and find the love of my life and get married happily for ever with all my sexual needs met for life?" My second cousin in Paris married a blonde bartender. His sex life, and hers for that matter, seemed to be very active and hot. Then real life started to get to them which caused a nasty divorce in less than a year.

Right before I could arrive at the conclusion that I should not lose the chance of the life time for sexual delight and even that wife of the suture, I was suddenly reminded of the $300 to $400 figure for an hour of sex in Mustang Ranch.

"Maybe later on after I have worked for some time, and have saved money." Then to finalize this thought I told myself, "Bryce, you are not the type that goes to bordellos!"
Then I quickly rushed back to the bus and resumed my trip. Deprivation lingered and it lingered painfully that day and festered for years afterward.
The puzzling question would pop in my mind again and again, "Why I did not have enough courage and do the act! Was I too wise for this kind of stupidity? Or, was I too dumb to lose a big chance like this?" Then remorsefully blaming myself, I had the final thought that it was not worth. Even $200 for one hour of pleasures of flesh was enough to pay for one month of my apartment rent! Nevertheless that $200 was a lot of money to me then.

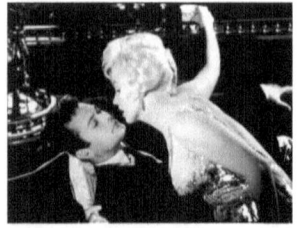

CHAPTER 10: French Upstairs Girls

In "Some Like it Hot" movie, Tony Curtis who is in love with Marylyn Monroe, one of the universally acclaimed sex symbols, tells her that "Not even French upstairs girls could excite him about sex." So, Marylyn kisses him romantically with the hope of reviving romantic desires of this rich and single man.

It turns out that when I was 26, I found one of these upstairs "salons" which was on top of a nice bar in Paris. The bartender would check from time to time to see who went upstairs. Generally it was OK to go to the private salon if you looked like a businessman, or if you were referred by a previous client.

This private salon had a small bar, with limited selection of drinks. The curtains were made of thick lavender velvet. There was a heavy scent of Chanel Number 5 mixed with fine cigarette smoke, and of scotch, Brandy, and Cognac.

Soft background music had some soothing effect. Some of the three of four tables were occupied by some of the most beautiful women. Each table was adorned by a small vase with fresh flowers in them. These vases reminded me of those in Van Gogh pictures. Everything in this room hinted of soft, supple, and intimate touch of a woman. In addition, this place was classy to the teeth.

As I paid more attention, I realized that one of these beauties gave a long passionate kiss to the gentleman who sat next to her. Some money changed hands, and then they went into one of the five or six small rooms that opened up to the salon and gently closed the door.

I felt a soft touch on my ear and then on my hair. Slowly, I turned around to see one of the sexiest women that I had ever seen in my life. She motioned me to join her for some Brandy. I could see her low cut blouse and was elated to see her cleavage. "You like these?" and then she looked at her breasts before her sentence was complete. She then quickly added, "Is Brandy OK?" The truth is that a sudden heavy surge of testosterone had made the choice of drink irrelevant.

Sipping Brandy right next to such desirable, sexy seductress of a woman was getting me even hotter. "Sixty Franks for half an hour, including the Brandy." She looked every bit like those manikins that one sees in high fashion stores and more. Manikins that had subliminally programmed my brain that this is all life is about. Gratification and satisfaction from intimacy, love, and sex with these women was the only sweet reward of life. In a New York second, I had given her seventy Franks that included a ten Frank tip, got up, and almost rushed her into a room.

Once I was totally satisfied, she lit a cigarette and offered me one too.

Before we were ready to return to the salon, she gave me another kiss and pressed her breasts against my chest. "I am from a good family from Lyon. My father left us when I was six, and my mother is not able to make ends meet. I have been doing this for eight years now. I have saved enough to buy her a Citroen. She spends two hours each day in the metro going from to work and back."

"Are you, an American?"She asked. Without waiting for my answer, she asked, "Yes. California?". I responded, "I wish I was from California. I am from Ohio." "Ohio, is that a province?" I told her that we had states instead of provinces. She seemed not to have heard of Ohio before, although French students normally get a heavy dose of geography. For some reason, they recognize Cincinnati as a famous American city when they hear it. Of course, this was before I moved to Chicago.

It is ironic that French tend to pronounce Cincinnati "Seen Sin Nutty!" You can interpret this any way you like.

As we were getting ready to leave the room, she noticed that I was still hard. She then gently pushed the door closed and said, here let me give you a bone voyage souvenir.

The souvenir was a quickie and several kisses accompanied by totally messing up of my hair in the process. "Here, give me your comb, let me comb your hair." "Sorry, I got over excited, and it is against the house rule to have any sex without payment. So, please keep this to yourself!"

The quickie however was more delightful and satisfying than the original act. She had not even bothered to undress after she had put on her dress. She took one of her tear shaped breasts out of its brassiere cup. Then she lifted her beautiful skirt with one hand. Then with her thumb she pushed her panty to the side while using other two fingers to open her vagina. Quickie lasted about six or seven minutes with both of us standing and her back against the wall.

To thank her I kissed her hand, European style, before we left our room. My deep, intense sexual gratification lasted several days. I felt like I was flying the next day and the day after that. I was a bit tired, but I was elated, revived, and felt that I was as good, as or even better than other men for having had sex with such beautiful hot woman.

She looked at her watch and whispered that she loved to see me again. In passing she told me that her next rendezvous should be there soon. In a few seconds, a very respectable business man in a nice suite and a Sulka tie came upstairs. Sulka ties were expensive and the height of fashion. They were distinctive and expensive.

I was telling myself that I was just as classy and as worthy of this upper class European for the fact that we had had sex with the same ultimate sexy woman that the entire Europe could offer.

Or, maybe, I was better. It seemed logical that the next client was a steady one who had been there many times before. To my pride and arrogance, she did not seem to be as passionate with him as she was with me. Furthermore, the overwhelming fact remains that she gave a wide and satisfied smile as she was pouring another Brandy for him.

The inherent envy in me as a man, almost forced me to one way or the other find out if he was given the quickie. Most likely not!

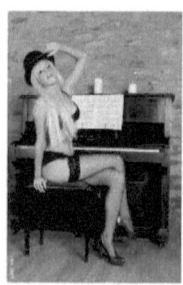

CHAPTER 11: Piano Teacher near Heathrow Airport

Rick Steves has been making fantastic European Travel TV shows for many years. He has a ten second fatherly advice in one of his programs. While showing some of the marvelous nude statues of bodies on public display in Rome, he adds, "Pursuit of pleasures of flesh always ends up in disappointment."

This was what I realized after my visit to see the piano teacher. Being single and an executive, I was getting all kind of advice from other colleagues. They introduced me to $1,000 suits from Nordstrom, tailor made shirts in Hong Kong, custom made shoes from Bally, and the piano teacher.

The piano teacher was originally an Air France flight attendant who would carefully select a few executive passengers in the First Class. Then she would be nice with them and take good care of them during the flight. Once she was sure that they were captivated with her beauty, culture, and manners, she would hint that she would be available for coffee.

Her tailor made navy blue uniform, airline supplied Parisian hair stylist, and classes on manners were irresistible.

This was her way of finding Mr. Right. She really wanted to get married. In fact, like me she really wanted to be happily married.

Unfortunately, after several months of dating these executives, and even non-executives, she came up with a depressive conclusion. These men were interested in one thing and one thing only! Typically, they wanted coffee on the first date, drinks on the second, and bed in the third and in that sequence. Then they would fade out or abruptly disappear on or before the fourth date.

Frustrated, she decided to help these hopeless and horny executive boys! During the coffee date, she would quickly decide if they are potentially husband material for her. If not, and if they seemed to have been captivated by her beauty, then she would tell them that her friend's apartment is available to her but she needs to pay rent.

Most of these playboys had no trouble understanding and paying the rent. Payment was almost always in cash and up in front so as not to be used as evidence.

She rented a nice apartment, or flat since that is what it is called in British English, and catered to carefully selected clients. However, there was a catch. She had to keep this legal. Therefore, she had a piano in the corner of the room and pretended that she was giving piano lessons.

Sure enough, she will always play and teach a few notes to the clients at the beginning, in the middle or at the end of the sex act.

I was told about this by a fellow business class traveler on a long flight to Japan. A few days before my next trip to London, I called the number and left a message that I was interested in my first Piano Lesson. Also, under the advice of my fellow business class traveler, I added that "Hans Licht" had referred me.

Got a nice call back and the day and time of the appointment were set. I arrived at the door a few minutes early. I rang the door bell, and the door opened. It was a goddess in hot pants who opened the door. "You must be Bryce, friend of Hans!" After she had made a nice drink, she took my coat and tie off to relax. Then, there were a few notes that she played. Then flaunting her astonishingly shapely breasts, she move to the bed and sat there. "We have a special that Hans likes. Would you be interested in that?" I felt rockets going off in my pants. Fireworks had already started and rockets were soon able to crash through the zipper and break through the zipper. Without knowing the details of Hans's special I nodded that that was what I liked to. OK, you want a half and half which is about $400.

Well, Hans in spite of his sexual interests that I was going to soon find out was a kind man. He had told me that I need to bargain, or negotiate, about the price. We settled at $250. I was proud of my negotiation skills. I think Herb Cohen who wrote the book on negotiations can be proud of me as well. In a blink of an eye, she was totally nude. At least that was how she looked to me. But legally she was not! She had left her ankle bracelet on. This would provide her with the technicality she needed not to get a fine if she was arrested for solicitation! She inspected me carefully to make sure I did not have any sexually transmittable disease. The touch of her soft and cold hand was enough to send me to the orbit. "Wow, you are hard!" The fact is that those few seconds that her examination took were lingering mixture of torture, anticipation of sex, pleasure, and agony for me.

She quickly and professionally put on the condom, and started to give me one of the most satisfying oral sex that I ever had. She could anticipate what I liked and what I did not. My manhood almost starting to pulsate, she started the second half of the "Half and Half." As if reading my mind, she rode me for several minutes. Then, it was missionary position for a few minutes, then doggie style. Doggie style was when I exploded inside her.

The explosion was so hard that I had to quickly inspect the condom after use. The condom was OK, but it was so hot that it gently burned, and tingled the palm of my hand as I was looking at it. The ecstasy of having had perfect sex with the perfect sex goddess had made me look and feel poetically world class romantic. I noticed the condom had a gold color that would almost become light purple as I held it up against the cold winter cloudy London skies just outside her window. As I was leaving after having been totally satisfied, I gave her a nice and long hug.

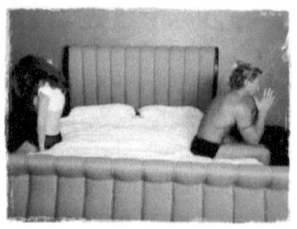 CHAPTER 12: No Woman Really and Honestly Likes Sex

The flip side of this question is the implied subtitle of the book: Do men ever get enough sex?

These are complicated, controversial, and even dangerous questions. I had tried to come up with some sort of peace with these two questions for myself. Not being a psychologist, or some sort of expert, the best I could do was to write down my experience in this book. This book is based on some notes that I had taken during my visit to the Red Light District. Furthermore, since it was written when I was in my late twenties and at the height of the sexual revolution, I was sure that these notes will shed some light on my question.

I was not disappointed; there was a lot of insight in these notes and thoughts.

Regarding the first question, it seemed that I would put my best foot forward, date woman and hope to impress them. Then second date, or third or fourth, hope that sex would naturally happen. Again, please do not forget that those were the days of sexual revolution.

My unwritten contract with myself was that I would remain a gentleman. I would do the right things and then let the women decided how far they wanted it to go. I did respect that.

This gave me enormous power and confidence. I never pushed and never begged. This strategy had made it possible for me to ask women out and usually get a favorable response. I seemed to enjoy a gentleman reputation among the members of the opposite sex.

I always said and did the things that I was expected to do to please my dates. I had many dates that I enjoyed beyond any imagination. If there was something that was better than sex, I had found it; it was in being trusted, liked, and enjoyed by women.

It is apparent that many of my dates also realized that life is just too short and let us enjoy this moment that we have together. I had become a conversationalist. I knew and had read enough about anything so I could carry an interesting conversation.

I had also learned to be genuinely and honestly interested in these women. It seemed simple to me; it was only human to be interested in another human's feelings, ambitions, fears, and thoughts.

However, being a man, and not getting enough sex, started to bother me. Was I failing? Was there a magic formula that everyone else knew and I did not? How come everyone else seemed to have more sex than I did? The fact is that most of the time I was not getting any.

As disappointments piled up, the best way that I could handle these was to think that women really do not like sex. It is sexist, chauvinist, stereotypical, one-sided, and whatever other negative adjective that you want to attach to it.

The irony is that this worked for me for years. It helped me keep my sanity. This desire dream of perfect sex was what helped me cope with life's harsh realities and Chicago's heartless and cold windy winters.

I would go into the first date assuming that there will be no closeness of any kind. Furthermore since ninety-nine percent of time there would be no such thing, then my expectations were not hurting me later on.

I expected nothing, and I got nothing and that was even and fair.

Shockingly, these notes that were written when I had saturation sex were telling me another story. At first, I thought someone might have written them since they did not quite add up to what I thought they should have. "Come on Bryce, who would have the time, or even care to spend time on your nonsense? M, .It is you, it is your handwriting and the stationary is from Temmel hotel in Amsterdam!" These thought convinced me to try to understand the notes deeper. I was satisfied to the limit with whatever sexual gratification is all about. At the moment of writing those notes, I had the opposite problem of Dean Martin. Dean Martin would look at attractive women and he would die to know how they looked in their panties or nude. He just had to see that. The urge was overwhelming. In addition, it did not mean anything how much he seen such women undress and become nude right in front of his eyes. He was dying to see the next one. He had to see them all nude!

Please let me explain what I mean by having the opposite of Dean Martin's problem.

Unlike him, I had seen so many most beautiful and sexy women nude, and had sex with them, that I was dying to see how they would look like with their dress on. Interestingly enough, this overpowering urge would not stop there. I would die to have a conversation with them; a human to human conversation. I would wonder how it would have felt had we been in love, rather than just in lust!

In my mind, I was wondering how it would feel if I was allowed to kiss them on the lips as their real lovers did. I was wondering how it would have felt if I would comb their hair or to give them hope and comfort as a lover does to a real lover.

I wonder if they had ever been married, or if they had had children. I wonder if we would have been innocent playmates when we were five or six year olds.

A therapist one time told me "Mr. Bryce, it is quite arrogant of you to compare yourself with Dean Martin or any other celebrities! In case you have forgotten, you are nothing!"

Speaking of innocent playmates, I must tell you this story. One time when I was on a business trip, I noticed that my wife was standing in the arrival area. She had a nice dress and a clean makeup. But I was totally surprised and shocked. I had not expected to see her in Denver. Of course, since our communication had broken down ages ago, I tried to make a good thing out of this. I said "What a surprise to see you here! What are you doing here in Denver?" "Well I am here on business too." Then without any further ado, she asked "Are you staying at Hyatt Regency? Did you have any checked in luggage?" Since the answer to both was no, she issued one of those "Follow me" orders that had to be obeyed or else all hell would break loose!

Somewhat hungry, jetlagged from the long flight from Heathrow, and under the weather because Denver is a mile high and my heart condition gets worst, I had no choice but to follow her.

"I used some of your frequent millage points to upgrade your room to a bridal suite" was all she told me on that twenty minute ride and she made it clear that she did not expect any answers or protests! I was a done deal. It was an act already completed and that was that! Any insubordinations would have not been tolerated. Not even from an antiwar activist like myself!

I was wondering why bridal?

I answered my own question by saying to myself "Bryce it is OK, you do not really need to make love to her. This is just because you snore and she wants a big room so she gets some sleep!" A pleasant thought like this did really put my mind at ease.

I asked her if she wanted to have a simple dinner before we went upstairs. Like a woman on a mission, she said "No, I am not hungry, plus I do not have time for that!" Then she showed a side of hers that I had seldom seen before. Instead of ordering me to follow her to the room, she said "You can have a dinner here if you spend no more than twenty minutes!"

As I entered the room I noticed that she was in bed. The next command was issued before I even took off my jacket and tie. "Me, you, have sex now!"

I failed and failed miserably. No sex!

When she realized nothing is going to happen, her next order was "Go get yourself a separate room!" It was a good thing that I had not taken my jacket off yet. I took my carryon baggage, and went to the desk!

The receptionist was a younger guy. Without asking any questions, or making it more embarrassing, he informed that there were no adjacent rooms available to where my wife was. "In fact Sir, there are no rooms available on that floor!" This was indeed good news to me!

Next day right about the time that my wife usually wakes up I knocked on her door. There was no answer. The receptionist told me that she had checked out at 7:00 AM to catch a flight back to Chicago! I was really puzzled. She had flown to Chicago just to spend a night and have sex with me? Something did not make sense! Something was cooking. She had come all the way to Denver to have sex with me in a hotel room? But we sleep on the same bed every night. All she had to do was to rollover and give me a kiss. Had she given me a passionate kiss that would have ignited my desires for sex, I had been like a powder keg of explosives. These are long term unsatisfied sexual stress caused by deprivation after marriage. I was hurt and confused. Did she really want to have sex with me out of desire or obligation? Is she as deprived as I am? Back to my old question; do women ever want sex?

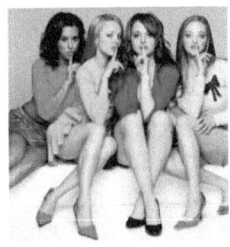 CHAPTER 13: Five Types of Women

When I fell in love with Roya, and in those long discussions we had, we had an idealistic and simplistic view of life and the world.

Roya and I really wanted to get married, become moms and dads, and forever live happily ever after playing house! Many years later, after I had become best friends with Diana, she had a different classification of women. Diana was introduced to me by a dating agency that charged a lot of money.

Diana's idea was clear. There were only five types of women in this world:

1. China Dolls,
2. Mothers,
3. Nurses,
4. Soul mates,
5. Intimate partners.

The China Dolls were those who were narcissistic about their looks. All in this category spent a lot of time in gyms for endless hours to keep their bodies great.

Mothers are those who will act as your wife and mother and take care of until there are children. With children, they would do their best to be a good mom. They would do this even if this mothering costs them their look, their marriage, or anything else.

My mind drifted to my own marriage. At the age fifty-eight, I was in a less than a perfect marriage. However, I had done the right thing by selecting the woman that I had married. If the stereotyping here was right, then I wanted to have a mother type.

Sure enough that was true. What had attracted me to my wife was the fact that as a babysitter, the kids that she was taking care of preferred to go to her rather than their own mom. She seemed to have a way with kids.

With these thoughts mingling in my mind, I seemed to have found a deep answer to a question regarding my own marriage.

Nurses are those who like to fix you and make you healthy. Soul mates are those who will spend a lot of time trying to understand you. They would spend hours and hours talking to you about your feelings or your childhood hurts or other subjects.

These are two people to fall in love, or lust, and have great sex together even if there is nothing else in common.

"Diana, this is stereotyping!" She quickly responded no, it was not! "This is a general idea about different women and what makes them do what they do." As I had expected, there was more to this, "As you can see, lover boy, you cannot have it all!" "You have to decide what is important to you. I mean that one thing and nothing more. If sex is what you want, then that is what you want. Do not expect intimacy, or motherhood, or other things. However, keep in mind that the woman that you can have the best sex with is usually not the one that is most attractive, unless you live on a Hollywood cinema screen! "

I am sure that there is also a comparable stereotyping for men as well. Unfortunately, I am ignorant about it.

I was puzzled by sex being one of those categorizations. But it did not take long before I remembered a second cousin who lives in Santa Barbara. He is handsome guy and as far as I remember he was always surrounded by attractive women. He proposed, and proposed in bed, to Irene after having known her for less than one month. They were crazy about each other, at least sexually. They were hoping for marriage to be a permanent honeymoon.

Divorce happened soon after marriage. This divorce broke both their hearts and their parent's heart too. They were love birds. How could this happen? No one could really answer. One day some time after the divorce, my cousin decided to tell me some details.

He did love Irene all right, but he lost interest after a few weeks, or a month or so. "I really did not want a relationship forever; I just was so lost in her beauty that I could not help myself. Once we both had our fill of romantic, idealized sex, and love for that matter, there was time for both of us to move away. We always moved away!"

The trill was in the chase!

I visited him and his parents, some years later in Paramus, New Jersey. He insisted that we go to the Miss USA Pageant Primaries that were held there. He had met one of the contestants before, and he really wanted to go to the pageant. Helga, the girl that he knew, looked even more attractive than ever before. She had an older sister, Sonia that was just as pretty. Before I know my cousin and Sonia disappeared. They were gone for about two hours and they returned just in time before the show was finished.

Sonia quickly announced that they had plans to get married. "What after two hours? Cousin, what happened?" His response was interesting. "We have a lot in common, and we had great sex in the back seat of the car. What else is there?" Then they dropped me in the bus station and they went to his apartment.

Almost eight months after that day they had twin boys. They got married soon after wards. They lived together until their boys were eighteen and then they split!

"We had excellent sex, and I was totally fulfilled. I am almost sure that she was also fulfilled too. Then, we had a problem each time we saw someone else that was attractive. We decided to have open marriage. We tried going to bed with other couples. Then we started to drift apart. Or maybe there was nothing to start with." He offered me some cold drink or the other and then continued. "Living with her was unbearable, he said. He also added something interesting. Even after their split, every time they met, if it was possible, they would have hot sex to release stress first. Bryce we were so great in bed, but we had nothing else in common!"

I had firsthand experience, and I perfectly understood what he was saying.

The thrill of search make you chase what is or seems impossible to catch. As one of my lovers told me, this is like a dog that chases a truck. If you cannot catch the truck, then you as man can console yourself in telling yourself, "Well she was not that great after all." This is the sour grapes syndrome.

But, there were several women that I fell for and succeeded to have an intimate relation with. Then, the "Blonde Blues" syndrome hit me.

Let me back up a bit.

We all know what refined and processed sugar is. However, the origin of this sugar is not known that well. In "Sugar Blues" which is a fantastic book about sugar, the history of sugar is carefully explained.

Sugar was originally so difficult and expensive to produce that only kings and emperors could have it. Then, since human bodies at that time were not used to this foreign substance, sugar would give them a high. This is similar to the same high that you can sometimes see in kids even today. When they eat something sugary, they become hyperactive and excited. This is part of human reaction similar to the high that heroin and cocaine produce.

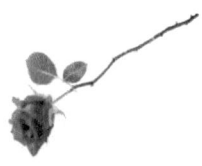 After this period of high, then there is a period of sudden and deep down, depression that ensues with sugar just like it does with drugs. This depression and low state is what the "Sugar Blues" is talking about as the blues.

When I was single, many times being intimate and especially having sex with a gorgeous woman would induce a high. Then as that high subsided and as time went on, I would lose interest.

This is what several of my partners have told me that this has happened to them too. Apparently, unlike many other stupid "man things" this can also affect smart women too.

In one case, I had found a total stranger, but extremely attractive woman in a meeting. After doing my refined eye contact and approach, I invited her for a drink. After the drink, we soon ended up in her apartment. With my cloths and her dress all over the bed room, we had some of the most exciting sex imaginable.

Then after we were done, she went to the kitchen and brought us cold drinks. Then I started to notice that she was not perfect. Without her high-heel shoes, she looked shorter that I had wanted to see her. As if she was reading my mind, she echoed, "Yeah, I am shorter!"

Then as we were leaving the apartment, she told me that if we are to make love again, she will insist that I keep my shirt and tie on "because it was the white shirt and the tie that turned her on!" At that moment, making love to her seemed not to be in my top list of the things to do.

We had done the chase, we had fulfilled our dreams, had our fun, and now this chapter was done and it was time for the next chapter.

A British comedy aired by the Public TV Channel named "Coupling" was full of these "One Night Stands" that always seemed to have the same alcoholic like behavior.

Speaking of British comedy, my wife had decided last year to do something about our lack of sex in our lives. At least that has been my working assumption. So, one day she called me and asked me to meet her for lunch in a prestigious health spa that also had nice massage and saunas. Her orders were, "Be there by 11:15 the latest and I see you in their restaurant. This restaurant overlooks Chicago River and is really nice. I was there even a few minutes earlier and managed to get a table. I noticed my wife arrived and she went directly to the manager. She told him something, and then she came directly to our table and told me, "Get up!" I had just started drinking my glass of Merlot. Before I could say anything, her instructions were, "Pay for it and bring it with you! Hurry up! I do not have all day! Come on get up and let us go!" I noticed she had a shopping bag full of stuff.

With great embarrassment, I followed her out of the restaurant and rushed out as if some emergency had happened. "Credit Card!" she demanded! "Yes Sir!" I replied and gave her my Visa Platinum!

Minutes later we were in the hot pool and sauna that had the threatening name of "Honeymooners". We undressed and we went into the hot water.

Well, nothing, absolutely nothing, happened in the Honeymooners Sauna room!

My wife was angry and disappointed. She did not speak a word. She put on her cloths and left without saying a word. It is things like this that turn me off and destroy any desires I might have for her. She could be the prettiest China doll, or the most loving mothers, or the sexiest caring nurses, the most affectionate and desirable soul mates, or the most magnetic intimate partners, but when she does these rage full things, I feel dejected!

I think that my wife has the rage version of alcoholism! She is always angry, or actually in rage about something or other. Her favorite saying is that the day after our divorce becomes final she will be the happiest woman on earth. I do not believe this. This is exactly what an alcoholic repeatedly tells himself!

The alcoholic says to himself, "I can stop drinking any time I want. But, I need to have just one more drink. Maybe this time I get the joy and satisfaction that I need to get from that next drink, and then I will stop. I will stop for sure then!"
Wrong, Wrong.
I was single for a long time, a very, very long time. As a matter of fact, I was single in the height of the sexual revolution. Everyone seemed to go to bed with everyone else. It is interesting that with all that sex, I could never find someone who had enough.
The trill was always in the next chase and as Abba the Swedish group says in a song, "To go get some more!"

CHAPTER 14: Men and Women

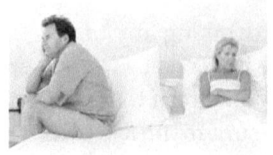

It is mind bugling that men think about sex almost every five minutes. Studies on whether women are the same or not is not conclusive.

First there is the rush to get some more. Then as my good friend Warren, the Limo Driver would say "The trill is in search!" I just heard over the radio that men get excited when they see images of nude women, but women get excited when they use their imagination while listening to words.

Women have sex to get intimacy. Men use intimacy to get sex. This in itself is somewhat of a perverted convoluted thing that evolution has brainwashed us to firmly believe in.

I remember the first time that I actually saw the picture of a totally nude woman was in high school. A classmate had dared to steal an X-rated magazine from his dad's office and bring it to the high school. Several of us were gathered around just admiring and going crazy about this work of beauty and art.

The first one to break the silence was a relatively stupid guy who commented, I had always wanted to know what a grown woman had under her panties. Now that I see it, it looks like it is just a crack. There is nothing in there. Why there is all this fuss?" That comment triggered a wise remark from another guy, "Well, because this tiny crack can make us guys feel in heaven!"

Another guy was trying to touch the genitals in the picture. As if trying to feel its softness or enjoy that touching sensation.

Another one is a very thoughtful way asked "I wonder if she is a natural blonde." That was when I could not stop showing off my superior intelligence. "Well, she is totally shaved and creamed and powdered down there, otherwise, we could tell if she was a natural blonde by the color of her pubic hair!" Then I decided to shut up my mouth since my erection was beginning to show in my pants.

About that time, another guy being totally amazed by this visual excitation had to chime in. He asked, "Is this the Strawberry Blonde that they talk about?" Interesting enough nobody really knew. We all had thought that Strawberry Blonde was a shade of gold color hair. I learned the truth many years later that the term was invented by James Cagney describing his mother's hair color which was actually red.

Roya and I both had gotten all we knew about sex from American and French movies. We had seen the unreal images of beautiful movie stars in perfect surroundings and we had all seen the images of perfect love making.

The darn thing about it was that we never could actually see the physical act of love making and sex. Either the camera would cut to the next scene and show two satisfied adults engaged in some conversation still nude in bed, or some other God awful avoidance that made us being tortured by our imagination.

"For God sake let me see the actual things interacting!" was what I would have screamed in a theater showing X rated movies. Curiosity was killing me.

Paris in particular is a beautiful and sexy city to see. Pierre-Louis Colin, in his book, "Guide to Pretty Women of Paris" points out that the French women are not afraid to be beautiful; they are not ashamed; they are not offended to be watched.

This was true when I first visited Paris when I was a teenager, and this is true now. The entire city, even the building architecture has a sexy shape and color coordination that turns men on. I do know that this is crazy to write. But it is true. What is also equally true is that these beauties can only be seen, but not touched!

Unfortunately, the book is in French and therefore difficult for Americans to understand and/or appreciate. Yet the fact remains that beauty is the same. The beauty in a flower is just the same beauty in pretty and well dressed men. As a man, I cannot say that I notice or care for beauty or handsomeness in men.

But, women, pretty or not need to be admired or even worshipped for their beauty on top of their humanity. Of course, people are people and they have to be respected for that fact in the first place.

In one of the comedy shows, there was a scene of a man who had finally managed to kiss and excite his girl friend and had managed to slowly and sensually undress her. The laughing matter was that he did not really know what to do next. He had never in his life gotten to that point. The woman who was somewhat older and therefore somewhat more experienced, had decided to be "proper" and pretend that she did not know what to do either. Then scene closed with the woman saying she had to go.

There was some laughter in the movie. But, I hated it. I did not really know what to do either. My education had had a big gap. The darn movies either used a sheet as the cover for the real sexual action, or they just drifted away, so I had never seen how it was to be done.

Some years later I arrived at a sad conclusion. The conclusion was that we and the society have wasted sex and intimacy. This loss is not only for singles but also for married ones as well. Our sex education has failed to teach us, even under the strictest ethical rules that sex and intimacy are important to human condition.

We need love to live.

Love in all its manifestations; Love as in caring for someone else; Love as in the physical art of having sex; Love as in closeness and intimacy; Love as in holding hands ; Love as in procreation; Love as in men getting rid of the urge while loving and satisfying in the proper way their loved ones and hopefully in marriage.

Back to that X rated magazine. It was discovered by the Principal and the guy who had brought it to school was expelled for three days. I just hate to think what that must have done to that guy's sexual life for the rest of his life.

One of my second cousins who lives in Europe and who is from a well to do family told me that in their sex education class one of their trusted and favorite teacher made an observation. His observation was that when his son becomes about sixteen; he plans to take him to one of the high class and clean and healthy bordellos in Paris. His idea was that this will be the right and safe way for his son to feel sexual pleasures and therefore not to go through the tortures of longing. Longing and not knowing what it feels like to satisfy a woman. Longing to know what it feels to be satisfied. This would also save his son from feeling depressingly deprived with a lot of pent up passion and desires to be as good as the next man when it came to sex and love.

He was quite ahead of his colleagues in this. Nevertheless, he does have a point. If it is experienced just once, then men and women will be better able to relate with each others. They then can become better soul mates.

They can become better soul mates by being better soul mates without the anguish of sexual stress and frustration. In fact one of my most trusted friends told me about his son who had to be hospitalized in a mental hospital since he could not control his sexual urges. This urge compelled him to having unprotected sex with two or three totally anonymous partners each day. Even with that he never felt totally satisfied. The more he got, the more he wanted to have.

I do know this well. A few months after my diagnosis I had to go to a business trip to Paris. This was a big show and tell about our next generation products. The sad part was that all these products will go to market about a few months after my death.

A few hours after my arrival on an Air France Concorde supersonic jetliner, I was sitting in my hotel room looking outside. It was a beautiful Paris afternoon in early May. Obviously, I had just missed the perfect April month which is the time of romance in Paris. Directly across the street, there was a flower shop that seemed to be owned by an elegant and strikingly attractive French black woman. She had just sold some flowers to a young and romantic man that her husband arrived. He too was a handsome and tall French black man with a very nice jacket and tie. They kissed for just over a minute while his hand gently found its way under her skirt and it went up her thy. As his hand was gently and romantically caressing her, they resumed their kissing. From a distance I could easily convince myself that he was tactfully, yet gently and slowly pulling down her panties. After all, this was Paris and the city of lovers. As this was going on in the daylight on a balmy day, I noticed that his hand was gently coming down on her ties and a few seconds later her panties fell on the floor with her feet still in it. I noticed her beautiful high heel shoes while she was gingerly maneuvering her feet out of the panties. Then they stopped kissing long enough so she can pick up the panties and hand it to the man. The man took a quick look around and quickly stuffed the panties in his leather jacket pocket.

I was hot! I was so hot that I could barely breathe. I felt like I had a fever. I would have given anything to be that man and in love with that woman. Her beige colored skirt strongly reminded me of Laura. Laura was my soul mate, lover, and confident some twenty years before this. I was indeed in love with her. Unfortunately, we were both too young then and we gradually drifted away from each other. I had tried many times to find her before. Unfortunately all of those attempts were unsuccessful. This time a mutual friend told me tht she had moved to Paris shortly after we had drifted apart. Since I had fantasized and missed her all these years, this time I was determined to find her.

Laura and I had a very hot and special love affair. Just like an angel, she had appeared in my life shortly after I was dumped by my girlfriend of several years. Laura, who was studying to get a doctoral degree in psychology from Sorbonne University, had gotten extremely interested in me. Our first meeting over a cup of coffee had lasted more than two hours. We shared our life story, our ambitions, and our sentimental and romantic ideals as if we had known each other for ages.

As the closing time arrived on this café, which is only a few metro stops away from Sorbonne, we left regretfully. To be a gentleman, I told her that I would like to walk her to her car. Right after we exited the café, our discussion somehow focused on intimacy. Since she had gained my total trust, I shared that "I have never had enough love intimacy, closeness, or for that matter sex!" She stopped walking. As a future psychologist, she was totally absorbed for trying to find why and how. She was genuinely interested and she cared.

By then we had arrived at her car. It was a black Renault. As it is customary at the end of a date, I asked her if I may kiss her. She did not say yes or no, but she gently tilted her head as if to say she was ready for a kiss. It was a somewhat stressful and shy kiss. Nevertheless, I somehow felt like she was hot too. After that we said goodbye and went our ways.

That night, I could not sleep. I was dreaming of a life time of love, sex, and marriage. It seemed that I had found my soul mate and it was Laura. However, there was one major problem. She was from an upper class family and unbelievably attractive. In addition, she was so intelligent that put her way above my league. Over a nice breakfast, I had convinced myself that I will never see her again. This was a painful conclusion that I would not accept. I knew her first name, and I knew she was in Sorbonne and in the psychology department. After a little detective work, I was dialing her number.

"Bryce, is that you? How did you find my phone number? Mon Dieu, I am so pleasantly surprised. Come, come, let us have a glass of wine in my tiny apartment. Where are you? I will come pick you up." Shortly after this, her black Renault stopped outside my hotel. She was driving so fast that there was some rubber mark on the street after she had jammed the brakes. She quickly opened the door and I could see her beautiful long legs since I was upstairs in the hotel looking down. As her beautiful legs touched the street level, she pulled her skirt up to adjust her pantyhose by pulling it up. I got a very short glimpse of her white and creamy velvet panties under the pantyhose. My heart stopped. However, she was not done yet. She opened her purse and took out a lipstick and freshened up while her skirt went up again. This time, I could have another glimpse of her panties. It was my dream to reach out and touch her beautiful and sexy panties.

After we had a glass of wine in the bar on the first floor of the hotel, she offered to give me a tour of Paris. Some sightseeing followed all the time that I just wanted to kiss her. "Stop, please stop!" I said. "What is wrong?" I immediately answered her that I could not take it. I was captivated by her friendship and beauty and I asked if I may kiss her again as I could not wait any more. "No! Not now!" Then she stopped the car in some parking lot that was hidden behind a restaurant. Then she declared, "You can kiss me anywhere now!" A long kiss followed that made both of us crazy about sex. By then my shyness struck me and struck me hard. Sensing this, she pulled her panties and pantyhose down enough so I can see her beautifully shaved pussy. "Do you like to just watch or do you want to touch too?" In matter of seconds my two fingers had found their way inside her while we were busy kissing. She then gently asked me to open my zipper. I did that and spread my legs a bit too. Her soft and beautiful hand was holding me sensually. Our passionate kisses had made the windows fog.

I felt the gentle movement of her hand while she was holding me that was in concert with my movement of my two fingers inside her. She then looked around carefully and without totally taking off her bra, she pulled one gorgeous breast out. I could sense that she had powdered her breast with some foundation powder. This foundation powder looked like microscopic bits of gold that shined on her purely white and blonde complexion. Her breast would almost glimmer or shimmer even though there was not much direct sunlight on it. Her nipple found its way into my mouth and I was going crazy.

I pulled down the back of my seat. This was nice since it went all the way down. She pulled down her skirt without pulling up her pantyhose and quickly got out of the driver seat. Then she horridly circled the car and came to my side. I had just barely put on the condom that she was on top of me and aligning herself so I could penetrate her more effortlessly.

"Oh my God, you are thick and hard! I love the way you move it inside me. It slides without much effort.'

After a most satisfying sex, we were both exhausted but ultimately satisfied. I used some of the Kleenex that was on top of her dashboard to clean her up. I was busy doing this when she started to do a touch up on her lipstick. This ignited my passion again. She had no problem reading my mind. "Do you want to do something crazy but extremely sexy?" Then as if to help explain, she added, "Last time I was on top. This time we will do it standing up. I make sure there is no pain in your back. Do you want to do this? You will love it and like it!" I had to remind her again and say that I have a bad back. "No problem!" She then got out of the passenger side and motioned me to get out too. With her back to the car and leaning on it, she lifted the front of her skirt and took my erect penis and effortlessly slid it inside her. I thought for a second about finding the other condom that I had in my other pocket. But I was not going to disrupt this once in a lifetime spontaneous sizzling hot sex!

I was just about ready to explode inside her when the owner of a beat up Citroen entered the parking lot and went towards his car. I have no doubt that he knew what we were doing. He seemed to be a nicely dressed and clean middle class man. In fact he looked like he was a professional like an attorney, or a teacher, or even a doctor. I started to panic as it seemed like he was walking towards us with a big and assuring smile on his face. I was scared all right, but I would not pull out of her if my life depended on it. We were still trying to complete our standing up sex near the car.

By now the man was about one foot away from both of us. I was still inside and with a big erection. Right about then I lost control. Just to make sure that I will not lose my stiff erection inside one of France's most beautiful women, I pulled almost all out and then I trusted my entire 17 Centimeters back inside her. She then went out of control and she let out a tiny scream of joy. At that moment, the unwritten contract between me, and these two French citizens seemed to be cast in concrete. The third man just wanted to watch and this made both of us much hornier. While Laura was looking me into the eyes as if to see if it was OK with me, she turned slightly around so the man could see better. She then pulled up her skirt and the man could delightfully see my fully erect penis insider her. He then asked, "May I?" Laura was quick to say "Yes, but a little touch in French!" He then gently and caringly looked at me to make sure it was OK with me too. He then pulled his hand out of his pants pocket and started to caress her with big care not to touch me. His hands were cold compared to sizzling heat on Laura and my body. Then he gave a relatively long kiss to her, gently touched her breast that was still out. Then he started to continue walking towards his parked car right after dusting off some of the powder on her breast, and licking the lipstick off his lips that was smeared by Laura's lip.

He was not even one step away that we both exploded in a strong ejaculation together. I was feeling her come on me and she was going crazy and horny with my rich and big come inside her.

This was now about eleven hours before my flight back home. I felt double time pressure; one was far more serious and it was for my limited remaining life, the other was for not missing that flight. Laura knew about my deadlines and she offered to take me to the airport in time for my flight. Incidentally, due to time restrictions I had to fly to Vienna with a layover of two hours and then connect to my direct flight on Austrian Airline to New York JFK Airport. In New York, I had to go to La Guardia Airport for the New York to Chicago flight. Being early summer, this was the only way I could arrive in time for the annual stock holder's meeting in Chicago.

I forced my mind to stop worrying and wondering about the flights to Chicago and started to listen to Laura's car radio. This was a very popular song by Edith Piaf, a very famous French singer of the forty's and fifty's that said, "I have no regret about the past I have all these souvenirs." Then my head was being gradually moved to rest on Laura's shoulder. As my head was moving, I noticed a copy of Le Monde newspaper that was not even opened. Somehow, that unopened newspaper seemed to speak to me about my life. It was unopened and it was not enjoyed, yet it was directly destined to go to trash bins. This was similar to my soon expected death.

I had married a woman who did not know how to love. Being the adult child of alcoholic parents, she could not trust men. She had remained a victim and this had made it almost impossible for her to enjoy intimacy and sex. In contrast, Laura seemed to enjoy getting and giving intimacy, love, and sexual pleasures.

By now, my head had approached her shoulder and it was anchoring and landing gently and poetically on her shoulder. I was quietly, yet intensely enjoying the warmth and touch of her breast against my chest. Her faint smile seemed to OK that. A golden yet faint late afternoon sun was showering us. I noticed that Laura was now resting her head against mine.

Since she was a psychologist, she asked "Did you like this? I had not done this type of intensely pleasurable sex since college days! I loved it and enjoyed every bit of it!" The first half of her question sounded like a typical question a therapist would ask in a therapy session. But the other half which was a confession from her to me was very personal and moving. Therapists seldom would do this in a therapy session.

"I am an incest survivor!" she suddenly confessed to me. It took me quite a bit of time to figure out and sadly believe what she was saying. In my way of life, this was a crime. It must have been hell for her. However soon after those thoughts, I seemed to cling to the survivor part of her sentence. I was proud of her for not having let the wreckage of the past destroy her future. In fact, in my book she was a heroine. She had become a psychologist from one of the best universities to help other victims to survive.

"I am very sorry to hear this!" I said and really meant it from the bottom of my heart. There was a complete discussion of details and then she was jolted into realizing that I had a long flight ahead of me. At that point, she quickly pushed her breast fully back in her bra cup without moving my head a bit. This seemed to remind me that there was an end to this lovely romance session just like there was an end to my life coming soon. In my mind I could smell the stench of nursing homes and sights of dying in a hospital.

My thoughts were joyfully beginning to become sweet imaginations of a loving, intimate, and fulfilling sex with Laura: Daydreams of having had two kids together; Daydreams of a nice house and intellectual parties with friends and colleagues from around the world; Daydreams of being called honey by an affectionate, sexy, and attractive woman.

However the reality was different. I loved and was married to mother of my children who had started a fight over nothing in our honeymoon. The same fight and rage that had persisted all along our marriage. The anger that consisted on telling me "I hate you! I hope that you come back in a body bag!" when I was living the house for my business trip to Paris two days ago. In fact, it had not stopped there. As I was opening the door to get out of the house and enter the cold, dark, and frigid Chicago windy and stormy weather that day, she topped her "bonne voyage" wishes with loudly saying, "Be a man and give me a damn divorce!" She said this loud enough that the limousine driver could hear it as he was helping me with putting my luggage into the trunk of the limousine. This driver seldom talked and he had a stiff upper lip. Nevertheless seeing this scene he felt sorry enough to mumble something like, "It is OK sir, we all have our difficulties in life."

I was dying, and none of these made any difference any more. Laura was driving to the hotel when the hourly news came on. AFP which is the official French news agency organization had several items to report including serious storms blanketing the entire Midwest with Chicago getting the brunt of it. The painful thoughts of storms and Diana's death wishes combined with the reality of dying seemed to try to persuade me not to return. I was wishfully thinking that if I stayed in Paris all these death and dying will not find me or get to me. In a rapid fire succession, Laura found and packed my clothes and things including a box of condoms. She gingerly inserted that box in between my shirts. We checked out from Grand Hotel Excelsior with a few minutes to spare from a hefty penalty for over staying.

"Laura, can we stop in Gallery La Fayette on our way? I have many memories of this place!" We were there soon. With six hours before the flight we decided to have a quick lunch or dinner at a café inside the gallery. Being absorbed in her beauty, somehow the words, "Laura, please marry me" insanely gushed out of my mouth echoing what I had felt for years in my heart with bypassing my brain. "We will have 'one of each' children, one boy and one girl; we go to symphonies, museums, concerts, lectures, and write books together!" Considering that I was 59 and she was 56, these words were in fact empty, hollow, and even idiotic. It was not just lust, it was real love.

Right before we left Gallery La Fayette, I had another request. "Can we go to the bridal dress section?" I asked her. She replied, "Honey anything that you want!" This was the place where Roya's wedding dress was supposed to come from. The wedding dress would have been symbol of an eternal love and a happy marriage for ever, and ever.

Unfortunately, that was the marriage that never happened. We were racing against time. Now I had about two hours and ten minutes left before I had to be in the airport. "Laura, can we go to the Notre Dame de Paris Church?" I wondered. "Honey, you can ask for the moon and I will get it for you!" was Laura's response without any hesitation. Once there, I got on my knees and prayed.

I found myself sinking deep in the stifling confinement of my seat number B3 with heartless engines noisily revving up to mercilessly leave Paris Airport. I was savoring a tiny taste and smudge of Laura's lipstick left on my lips after our last kiss. A few minutes after the seatbelt signs were turned off, a flight attendant gave me a single red long stemmed rose and said "Laura personally gave me this to give it to you." The stem had a tiny paper that said, "Produce of Israel" and a silver paper wrapped around a tiny water reservoir attached to the bottom of the stem so it is not denied of its nourishments and wilt. My concentration on the rose was disrupted by the flight attendant bringing a tiny envelope with the word Austrian Airlines embossed on it. Then with a gentle smile and dutifully, she said that they normally did not print emails for passengers. However, they made an exception this time since they thought you were newly married love birds and were separating from each other for the first time. French in general are poetically very sensitive to these matters of heart and romance.

The message inside which was a faint printout of an email said: "I loved every moment of being with you even though we were together for such a short time. I am sorry about things not working between you and Roya and that wedding dress from Gallery La Fayette. I promise to make it up to you on our next time together!" As poetical as the message was, it ended with a cold and computerized email address that read **laura_dps@surbonne.edu**.

The message helped me regain my thoughts of boundless joys and pleasures that we had had. As I was submerging again into my sorrow and agonizing pain of losing her again, my eyes got fixated on my tie. This was an elegant with gold, navy blue, and dark crimson stripes.

This was a nice blend of premier silk and Egyptian pure cotton and it was my favorite coloration. I guess the sparkling gold stripes reminded me of blondes. Furthermore, the velvet-like smooth touch lured me to deceive myself into believing that I was touching a lovely and sexy woman.

My expensive dress tie, being a Nordstrom classic, was made of linen and little combed cotton. This shirt was also gentle to the touch and color coordinated with the golden stripe on the tie. The color was an extremely light gold that reminded me of a natural blonde woman's sexy skin.

As I was admiring my tie, I noticed that there seemed to be a tiny smear of what looked like gold dust on the crimson stripe. Upon careful examination, this turned out to be a few specs of Laura's foundation powder that she had worn on her beautiful breast. This must have happened while I was resting my head on her shoulder and enjoying the touch of her breast that was outside the bra and against my chest.

My emotions burst into a flame just like gasoline touched by a torch. Then insanity prevailed. "Maybe I should talk to the flight attendant and tell her about my painful agony of being sexually aroused so bad that I needed some medication to cool down. Maybe the flight attendant will give me mouth to mouth resuscitation.

As the aircraft air-conditioning was turned full blast, I started to feel a chill going down my spine. I felt a deep sense of hopelessness combined with a heavy dose of despair.

This is extremely similar to what a drug addict or alcoholic feels for a love and sex addict. After all, healthy sex increases the production or Serotonin the same way that drugs do. And when this is not available, the shivering hands and hopelessness is the result. Please do not get me wrong, satisfying and fulfilling sex in a stable and responsible relationship is one of the nature's best gifts to us. It can enhance the relationship so much more. It is the irresponsible and sometimes violent sex that is the problem. It is the desire to have sex with all different women for once and then drop them that has consequences.

Just like a helpless alcoholic experiencing withdrawals, I was feeling the same cold and depressing feelings in my bones. It seemed that love, intimacy, communication, closeness, companionship, and sex had lifted me up to the top of the world. Then only a few minutes after giving her a hug and saying goodbye, I was hopelessly miserable; I was full or remorse; I was seriously thinking about taking the next flight back to Paris as soon as I arrived in Vienna. In **Out of the Shadows: Understanding Sexual Addiction** - Paperback by Patrick J. Carnes, he does explain the eerie, yet confounding, and strong resemblance between sex and love addiction and alcoholism. He also recommends the same twelve step of AA to be used in both cases.

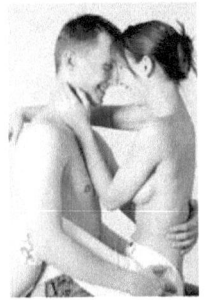 CHAPTER 15: Soul Mates

I think that unfortunately many Americans never benefit from having a soul mate at some point of their lives. Somehow, married or not, it never comes to trusting another person, especially a lover full hundred percent. It seems like they do not want emotions be tangled up with marriage and/or sex. I have seen men or women tell life secrets to other totally stranger fellow passengers in an airplane or in a bar. These are secrets that they never tell their loved ones or better haves, or marriage partners of twenty or more years.

Since I was single for the longest time, I learned how to be a soul mate, and I was extremely lucky to have several soul mates. One was a divorced woman whose ex-husband was even a communicative man who gave lectures to room full of management routinely. Her old husband loved her dearly and she loved him too. Unfortunately, they were not intimate and they were worried about discussing feelings. They were afraid that getting too close, especially is bad for marriage.

Somehow, she felt totally safe to talk about things with me. Marriage was never again an option for her. Even so, we both tended to enjoy a good conversation after a dinner. Surprising enough in the six or seven month that we saw each other, there was never any sex.

I trusted her so much, that I told her everything. The amazing thing about this is that once one tells another human being about our feelings, then a heavy weight is lifted from our shoulders.

I was also very lucky to meet Mary. She was a bank executive who was exceptionally pretty. She was very good at teasing men. In fact, in our first date, our discussion of general things quickly gave way to sharing our thoughts about sex. To my surprise, she suddenly switched topics and stopped pretending that she was flirting with me.

Several dates later, she told me that she goes through the emotions, and she pretends, but she is too hurt to have any joy or excitement about intimacy. As her depression got worse, she started to intentionally look less desirable, pretty, or sexy. Instead of buying and wearing the most stylish clothes from Macy's or Nordstrom, she would wear clothes on sale from less glamorous stores. If the sales woman told her that she looked great in a dress, she would intentionally not buy that one.

Her beauty had caused her serious grief. She had spent many of her life with men who were not really interested in her as a human being, but in her as a sex object. Thus, she had developed this life saving strategy of teasing men in the first or second date. If they did not have control and tried to go beyond her boundaries, then she knew they were not her type and she would drop them quickly.

She told me I was different, even though I was the same man as all the others. What was different with me was that she felt safe, and trusted me before the end of our first date.

Her glamour eroded steadily. Her joy and smile disappeared with her wit and ability to be intimate with anyone. Then one day, as I was saying something, I noticed that tears raced down her face. These were cold tears. These tears were caused because she felt that she had done everything wrong in her life. Tears that in spite her education and financial success made her feel like a complete loser. She wanted a happy home and children. But she would never have that. I asked her why. She said it was too late.

As a child she had witnessed how her alcoholic father beat her mother. She had felt sorry for her mother who had nowhere to go. She also bitterly remembered that her father would normally call her mother most terrible names, and then grab her hand and push her into the bedroom.

If this is intimacy and sex, Mary did not want any part of that. She told me that I was not that smart to go after glamorous women. She would tell me that these woman are "formulated such to destroy the life of people like you. Bryce, do not let this appearance deceive you. They are empty inside. They are spoiled by the society that worships their outside."

I had fallen for her.

Nonetheless, she was not going to be any more than a soul mate. She had made this very clear from the beginning. Slowly she started to push me away. Slowly, she decided to totally absorb herself in her work.

Several years later I bumped into this extremely obese woman whose voice I could clearly recognize. But, I could not remember who she was. "Bryce, this is Mary. I hope that you still remember me! Do you?" Slowly and painfully I realized this was Mary. Mary, one of the most elegant ladies I had ever met. This was the very same Mary who knew all the secrets in my life, and I knew all hers.

Similar to Mary, I had known a couple who were my friends before they got married and they remained so after marriage as well. From time to time we go to dinner in our favorite Italian restaurant in Chicago. We also loved to go to movies particularly on their opening night.

Bettina had always wanted to get married. We got introduced together during dinner in the university cafeteria by Larry. They were dating and they had plans to get married right after graduation.

They did get married. After living a few blocks from us in Chicago for several years, they decided to go back to Wisconsin and start their life there. Bettina had an alcoholic father and her mother was never close to her. Nevertheless, she was determined to make her own marriage a success. She sometimes talked about happy marriage instead of marriage. They started really nice, but a miscarriage made her go into severe depression.

Bettina was hurt immensely by this miscarriage. This would have been her first child. Also, according to her theories, children were fundamental part of a happy marriage! She had been determined to make a happy marriage unlike the miserable one that her parents had.

The miscarriage had happened due to her heavy dependency on prescription medications.

Larry had called me a few times telling me about this and then asking me what I would have done if I was in his place to face this calamity. As a friend, I did my best to calm him down. Give him some hope and tell him that things will get better. Somehow his calls stopped. I had left him a few voice mails, but he did not return my calls. Then, after several years, I got a call from Larry telling me that he had filed for divorce. He told me that things had gotten terribly bad between him and Bettina. In fact he suggested that I do not talk to her if she called. Luckily, or unluckily she did not call. As a matter of fact Larry did not call either. I took this in stride the best I knew. I knew that when divorce happens, some of the old friends and acquaintances of the old couple are shut out too. They tell me this is because the divorced couple now tries to make a new life.

I never, ever heard from Larry.

Most shockingly, I got a call from Bettina when she was visiting a relative in Chicago. I went to meet with her against my own best judgment. I offered to buy dinner and she accepted. I also invited her relative as well. As a rule, I prefer not to be alone with other women. Bettina paused for a second, and then told me that she will extend this invitation. But her relative most likely won't be able to come. Her clothing was faded, modest, yet still stylish. Her auburn hair was not shimmering as it had always been before.

My wife knew about this dinner arrangement. I had told her this will be a good idea for her to be there. Of course, I had no idea about what was going to be discussed. However, she had decided to not join us as she did not know Bettina or Larry as well as I knew them.

This was her most favorite Italian restaurant. The food was fantastic. Then she started to remember the first time that she had seen Larry. Soon she was telling me about the wedding day and their first child after miscarriage. Then, there was the first car they bought which was a beat up Ford Falcon, and right after that her sudden struggle with depression after her miscarriage and her mother passing away a few months after that.

Her father was abusive and violent. He was drunk most of the time. Her parent's marriage was hell. There never was enough money, food, or love. Speaking of love, the only thing that she remembers from her childhood is hate. Hate instead of love, was a survival mechanism. She learned this bitter lesson from her mom.

"Was Larry an alcoholic?" I asked. "No the bastard was not! I meant Larry. He also never touched drugs either." "So what happened? May I ask? Of course, it is not my business." "Oh well, the problem was not his, it was mine, but it is too late by then."

She decided to vent. "After many years of going to the Adult Children of Alcoholics, I have figured out what happened. I was getting revenge from my dad! Of course, I was seriously sick with depression."

"I made life miserable for the bastard. I figured out exactly how to piss him off and I did it every time. I pushed his buttons. When his boss called to tell me that he was being considered for a promotion, I told him that my husband should not be promoted. When the boss asked why, I told him that he beats me and children. Larry did not get that well deserved promotion that I knew he worked on for all these years. Then when he was going to Florida for some business trip, I made sure that he could never find some of the most critical documents that he had worked on for several weeks. Things got worse and worse and he got fired."

Bettina stopped for a moment and pulled out a picture of her and children from her bag. There were many smiles in this family picture from the happy days. Then, she quickly shoved that picture back into her bag and asked, "Where was I?"

"It was until my old son ended up in a foster home that I realized what was happening. My therapist had told me that I really needed medications to deal with my depression. So, I found a good Psychiatrist and I followed his prescription."

"I had managed to drive him to ground to get even with my dad. In the process everything else got worse and worse. Several times, he had to call the cops just to cool me down. I had also managed to get our kids to hate their own dad."

"I would withhold sex from him then I would tell my kids that your dad has no respect for me." Then as if a confession was coming out, she said, "I should have been jailed for all these!"

I cannot say that I was soul mate with Bettina. Yet, I was painfully beginning to understand what she was saying. Then, I had to ask my stupid question. I asked "Where is Larry?" Her answer with a big sorrow on her face was "He killed himself!" As soon as these words came out of her mouth, she tried to erase them. "I do not mean that he killed himself. He just did not take care of himself. His health got worse and worse as time went by. I did not care either."

By then my "dad is bad" campaign was in full swing. No matter how hard he tried, no matter what he did to recover the love of the kids, I did not let him. "I am now positive that this was what broke his heart and killed him. His own kids hated him! I lied to them and told them that dad had some money stashed away and he we too cheap to spend that for better food for the family. When he had his first heart attack, I ordered the kids to go to another room and watch TV. They were six and eight years old. They must have figured out what was happening, but my orders were strict. It was only after I saw his face red and struggling with breathing that I called the 911 Emergency." Years later when I was in the twelve step program, my older kid asked me if I was trying to kill my husband; their dad, even though everybody knew he was stupid and no good for nothing!

"What about the kids?" I asked. "Well, one is in a foster home that he has been for a long time and he does not talk to me. He does not even want to see me!" Then, with a smile, "As for my daughter she lives with me. I have told her the truth about Larry and I and she tells me that she has forgiven me."

I noticed that Bettina sometimes referred to her deceased husband as Larry and some other times as "Bastard."

She started to share more of some deeply painful memories. I knew that she respected and trusted me. "I had two friends who helped me immensely in this. One was my drug dealer. He looks and acts just like a normal person. He pretends that he worked in a law office. Yet most of his income is from selling legal and illegal drugs to people like me. As I was getting more and more addicted to these so called prescription drugs, he would ask for more and more money. When I was two months pregnant he offered to deliver my drugs to my home."

With an angry expression on her face, she added that "I should have never, ever accepted that. He brought the drugs and then asked if I could make him a cup of coffee. I did and he drank his and I drank mine. I do not remember much more after that until I woke up naked in my bed in my bedroom with scratches in my genital area and teeth marks on my breast. There was bleeding and I was too scared to go to a doctor." With her voice reflecting a lot of hurt and sorrow, she continued. "When I woke up, I realized that I was clumsily shaved too. Razor nicks, burns, and scratches could be seen in several places. He must have used Larry's razor blades. Suddenly, the idea that I was violated hit me between the eyes. I was still in the drug induced fog, but awake enough to try to figure out details. The eerie feeling that he must have inserted his stubby fingers with black fungal spores under them into me was nauseating and criminally abusive. This made me feel appalled, repulsed, and outraged. When I put my feet down on the carpet to go wash up, I felt his wet cold slippery seaman under my feet. I felt this eerie seaman on several spots. He must have had multiple orgasms and the sex was unprotected.

Somehow, I could not control my rage anymore. "Bettina, this is rape! This is a premeditated criminal act. This is an assault. This is like a murder. This is not sex. This is an act of violence." As I was uttering my serious objection trying to convince her of the severity of this cowardly act, I sensed that either she was not listening, or she for some reason did not wholeheartedly agree. She was looking down as if in shame, denial, or whatever the reason. Just to reiterate, I had to say one more time. "Bettina, this is criminal act! This is punishable by law and I hope that he gets the full extent of judicial vengeance!" I noticed that I was too irate to be rational. So, to cool myself down and give her one more reason, I added that "In French the word used for rape is viola! You guessed it. It comes from the word violence. No man or woman deserves to be raped as it is a savage, criminal act! No exception!"

I was feeling nauseated from these thoughts. " I asked "Why you did not call the police?" Her answer is an enigma until today. She mumbled something like "I hated it, it was painful, it was humiliating, and nevertheless I got some sort of sick perverted relief. It was as if my pent up sexual urges were sort of served with this savage violent act. I also felt that I deserved this punishment."

Observing my total disgust and feeling somewhat ashamed, apologetically she tried to explain. "You see, this is strange. I know. I betrayed my husband and our marriage. I accepted his invitation to come to my house. I am completely responsible for the miscarriage. But then, when it comes to sex, as a result of this experience, I think that I have become a different subhuman. I am different. I am painfully different. But this difference makes me feel, sense and fulfill my lustful sexual desires!"

Apparently, my emphatic argument that no one deserves to be violated by rape had fallen on deaf ears.

Being a man and having heard these things, my one track mind started to get active. In my mind's eye, I started to undress her. Then, I tried to imagine how she looked after having been shaved. I could not help but notice her extremely light complexion, her long fingers, and beautifully manicured fingernails. I was visually contrasting her beautifully manicured fingers as a symbol of feminine beauty with that beast's dirty and fungus infested fingers. As my desire for her was getting to boiling point, a hard stop like a ton of bricks hit me. The hard stop had been insinuated by my ethics regarding violence, crime, and law.

It was true that I was married. It was also true that I had not had sex for centuries. I felt big desires towards having sex with Bettina. The sex police in my mind issued a stern warning. The edict was clear "No sex with her, or affair, now or never is allowed outside marriage for you Bryce!" I was ethical, moral and I was faithful to my wife; a wife that did not look appealing to me; a wife who was always angry and belligerent; a wife that I loved, but was not attracted sensually to.

She had started to say something else while my mind had wondered and my imagination had gone wild. I collected my thoughts and focused on what she was saying. She was totally dependent on these drugs and each time he delivered, there was about an hour of rough sex. Later on, the dealer did not even have to use any date rape drug to get what he wanted. Bettina was attracted to this guy in a confusing, painful, and insane way. As if these things could not get any worse, the dealer would lecture Bettina each time after sex about how she had the right to destroy Larry, her husband. In a total convoluted and perverted way, Richard took pleasure in destroying Bettina's marriage and life. On one occasion he had even told Bettina that in the Bible, psalm 118 says that you have destroyed your enemies. And her husband was the enemy. There was no doubt. Of course, this was his interpretation to serve his criminal intent.

Bettina also had a sadistic girl friend whose name was Evelyn. She also had other serious psychological disorders as well. Bettina had become friends with Evelyn when they were both singles. They would go to single activities together. They were also both members of an expensive singles club. Bettina was lucky to find Larry quickly and really fall in love with him. Bettina had detected the fact that this was an honest and caring man. The fact was that Bettina had found someone and Evelyn had not. This made Evelyn envious. Evelyn was envious enough to sabotage the relation for Bettina. In addition to the drug dealer, Evelyn was instrumental in helping Bettina literally torture Larry.

It was starting to get late and I was really sad to hear what had happened to Larry.

On the way home, I started to have flash backs. "What would have my marriage been with Roya or Laura? Not that we were ever married, but would we have had fights or divorce?"

The fact is that I do know a real bastard of a husband. His name is Robert and he was my business partner for several years before he took most of our money and ran.

Robert is a good looking man from a bitter childhood from a broken family. His parents divorced when he was no more than nine. His step father used to beat his mother and his mother had one affair after another. Somehow Robert, a first class sales and marketing professional, was incapable of love. He had no sympathy for other human beings and he was extremely selfish.

Robert now reminds me of kids in a Romanian orphanage during the Chauchescu Dictatorship. These kids were so badly treated that they had developed a brutal and violent survival instinct. Of course, life was difficult for all then, but these particular kids exhibited the worse. They had no sympathy or empathy for other human beings. Worse of all, love did not mean anything to them. They just were not capable of any feelings, including love.

Robert had no time for his wife and family, but bars and gyms were his hangout. He always had his beloved gym bag in his car and he always went for his workouts. Soon he became an instructor and this was his way to meet and attract many most beautiful women.

Being a professional salesman he knew how to make women fall for him. One day I told him how jealous I was of his extreme popularity with the most attractive women. His response was, "Bryce, it takes a lot of work, experience, and excellent genes."

We hired him thinking he had an MBA degree from a reputable university back in the Northeast. It turned out that he was a college drop out in his sophomore year. He never finished up his college. Women were his obsession. He lived for Friday night dates. Saturdays, he usually had one of two dates. Ironically his Sundays were spent to recover from having too much "Sex and booze!"

No matter how much sex he had had during the weekend, by Monday, he was ready to launch his new chase to find the next woman. He would be going crazy for a woman sexually one minute and then as soon as something changed in her dress or makeup, he would lose interest. Then the chase was over and he had to find the next. There also was this insane characterization that he had. If he had had sex with a nurse, then he would not be interested in another nurse. He was constantly thinking that since this type of look, or career, had failed to "satisfy" him, he better go get some more of the other kind.

On a long flight from a difficult business trip he suddenly opened up to me after all those years. Of course, he was too drunk to care and the flight attendants had refused to give him more drinks by the. So, we had this stupid routine worked out in those situations. We both order the same drinks. And since we knew that his drink will have a lot less or no alcohol, we switched drinks as soon as the poor flight attendant was gone. This was sort of routine practice to keep passengers from becoming unruly during the flight.

At any rate, he then confessed of his most important rule. That rule was, "Never, ever, have sex with the same woman more than once. More importantly, if they even mentioned love, you should run just as fast as you can!"

However, he had been married for some years to an angle of a woman who wanted to have a "Father figure" for her lovely daughter. She worked hard to provide for Robert. She also had made the mistake of telling Robert that one night stands were OK for him to have. Robert has taken this to mean that he is free to have affairs by pretending that those are only one night stands. Robert feels no obligation, no commitment, and no ethics.

He does not wear a wedding ring and spends a lot of time in bars. He loves sports bars. Because of his looks he is able to pick up women almost regularly. Sadly, once the conquest is made, then he turns into this man who has no feelings and does not care. He tries to get out of that woman's life just as soon as possible. Even a few days are too long. He just wanted to be out, and never to see the woman again.

Some years ago, I had decided not to judge people. Nevertheless, I cannot ever sort out these two cases. I feel extremely sad for Robert's wife, and Larry.

Both my wife and I have been very close to divorce, many times in the past. That being the case, I had never really thought about the consequences on our children.

A few weeks ago, she got up from her bed and told me that she hates me. Then she went downstairs and started to cry. I had learned before that when this happens, I need the get the hell out of the house as soon as I can.

I slowly went downstairs, took my jacket and snuck out of the backdoor. I returned a few hours later. I could not help but hear that she was telling her best friend. She was saying, "Harriet, I love this stupid, stinky man. I gave him the best years of my life. Why is he doing these things to me?" "His Cardiologist told me that he does not have long to live!" "Without him, I would be lost!"

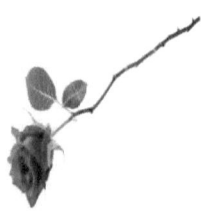

My wife, in spite all the faults that she continually found in me and all the arguments was a soul mate of the rough kind. Sometimes her verbal abuse will drive me crazy. However, one time she had clearly described to me that there was no such a thing as verbal abuse in marriage.

She and Harriet had bought and carefully read the book titled "Why Smart Women Marry Stupid Men?" As far as they were concerned, this book was precisely written for them and their marriages.

That day, I also heard her tell Harriet another one of her secrets. She admittedly said, "I do not know why, but I keep attacking this poor man! I give him hell regularly and he keeps coming back for more."

She is smart alright. She has a Masters degree in English. Unfortunately, she has never made a career out of her education. This might well be one reason she is so angry all the time. One of her secrets is that she really considers herself a failure because she had never managed to make a career out of her degree and expensive college education.

After being gone for two hours, and thinking that the coast was clear, I gently opened the door and entered the house. "You, good for nothing stupid man, I have had enough with you! You are as stupid at sixty as you were when I married you! You have wasted my life! God will get you for this." At least she did not threaten divorce that day!

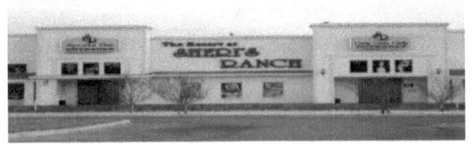

CHAPTER 16:
Sheri's Ranch

I came home one evening to see my wife of almost twenty years worried. "What happened? Why do you look so worried?"
"Your cardiologist's office called. That is what happened. Are you evading them?" I quickly realized that I had to deal with this, and deal with it swiftly. "No honey. Do not even think this way."
"Well the nurse told me this is the third time they have tried to find you. Apparently, you had refused to do a twenty-four hour heart monitor test and the Doctor wants to know why. "
Then raising her voice some and pointing her pencil at me, she said, "you can play Russian Roulette with your life all you want. But, I will not let you play with mine and your children!"
In my mind, I started to think about the Doctor and this most recent below the belt punch.
"Well I did not take the test because it is expensive. I did not take the test because even if the result shows that I have heart problems, what difference would that make. I am fifty-nine and at most I have three or four more years to live. So, I would be caught dead doing a high risk hear surgery, or implant a cadaver's spine disk in mine!" With some rage that was confined to me, I repeated the lyrics of Grace Slick of Jefferson Airplane. "You will not catch me lying face down!"
I wanted to take a picket sign and write on it "Hell I Won't Go!" as I did during the Vietnam War.
"I cannot hear you! What are you thinking? I am not a mind reader! Speak up. What is your game this time Mr. Condon, Mr. Bryce Condon?" Picket signs in my mind immediately melted away to the dungeons of history.

After years of marriage, we learn how to push each other's buttons. My wife had the upper hand in the judgmental choice of painful word combinations. Cannot hear you and what you are thinking implied that she as a wife was legally entitled to hearing what I was thinking. Her frustration was reflected in the usage of the "Speak up" part.

The red flag was is the double alarm usage of "Mr. Condon", which implied she was angry. Alarmingly usage of the "Mr. Bryce Condon" meant she had caught me in a capital offense and I was in serious trouble.

This trouble did not simply meant divorce. That was a repeated threat that had already worn out its impact on me. This could be a life threatening situation.

Use of powerful words is supposed to be my specialization as a writer and public speaker. Nevertheless, I admit that my wife is by far more powerful than I am.

The episode is not complete yet.

Standing right next to me, she said you will pay for this, and you will pay dearly. I do not care if you drop dead tomorrow. Do not take care of yourself. I do not care anymore.

Then just like a traffic cop that has stopped you for going fifty miles in a twenty-five mile zone, she grabbed my collar and seemed like she was going to whisper in my ear something. She had my ear, but whispering she was not. She was screaming so loud that my neighbors could hear.

"Mister, I let you off easy last time!" yanking my collar with a sharp pull, she showed me a bill for our daughter. The bill was from her dentist and it was for about $125.

"Among other things, this is overdue. Do you see the red sticker?" I admitted seeing the damning evidence like a sheep.

"OK Mister, write me a check. A check for $500 so I can pay this bill and plus the fines!"

"What? The bill is $125! Let me pay it!"

"No you had your chance, and you messed it up! This is just like you messed up this marriage!" Then as if she was going to give me a break, she said pay it up now before it gets worse."

"Before I could tell her that I did not have my checkbook, she picked it up from the table and put it into my hands. "Here write a check for $500!"

My six grader observing this the same way an intern observes the master, was standing there without a word. She was clearly not scared! In fact, she was convinced long time ago that "Us girls must stand together!" My daughter and my wife had black mailed me together many times!

"Write the $500 check!" she said. I asked if I could have my cell phone. The quick and short answer was "Why on earth you want your cell phone when you are supposed to write a check!" I quietly told her that I needed my cell phone to call the police.

"Stop joking write the check for $550!"

I wrote a check for $500! I had to prove my masculinity. Had I written it for the entire $550, even though it was for a $125 bill, I would have been a disgrace to my gender!

She grabbed the check and said "I asked for $550. This is only $500." I did not answer. With a semi smile on both their faces they went to the Mall. Interesting thing was that I could hear them right outside the door. My wife was telling my daughter, "See, I told you he will give in!"

There is a joke that I heard from one of my friends. The joke asks, "What is the difference between a spouse and a terrorist?" The answer is "You can always negotiate with the terrorist!"

This theatrical altercation, among many similar ones, is just like the "Honeymooners" show on TV ages ago. Jackie Gleason usually went on these rampages like my wife does. Yet, they loved each other and lived together even though this was not the happily ever after.

As soon as they had left, I got in front of my computer and did a comprehensive search for legal brothels.

The top among many was Sheri's Ranch which is an hour away from Las Vegas. One of the most amazing things about Las Vegas is that prostitution is illegal in Las Vegas. Difficult to believe, but it is true.

In spite the fact that prostitutes can be seen parading everywhere in the Casinos and on the Strip; in spite numerous handouts with pictures of nude women and address and phone numbers of prostitutes; in spite multitude of strikingly sexy and bikini clad women serving free drinks in the casinos, the law prohibits prostitutions in Las Vegas.

So, as a law abiding decent citizen Las Vegas was out of question for me.

Right below Sheri's Ranch, there was Chicken Ranch in the Google listing of the legal brothels. The word premiere was what caught my eye regarding Sheri's Ranch.

As I looked at their website, I noticed it was classy and in fact I could tell they were premier. I called the Las Vegas 702 area code number that was listed.

A nice, but sexy voice answered.

Before I could say much this woman, a total stranger, had read my mind before the end of my first question. She knew beyond a doubt that I was a first timer! "We are open 24/7 and we are a legal establishment registered by state of Nevada!" Then she carefully answered all my questions. She answered my questions as if it was the first time she had heard them. Of course, she must have heard these questions millions of times. "We are a clean establishment. Our ladies have to live on the premises and take the AIDS test. Our ladies are independent contractors, and they set their own prices." Then she told me that "You can negotiate the type of activity, and what you want to pay."

I thanked her and hung up. One thing stuck to my mind. "They had doctors checking their ladies regularly and no one has ever been infected by any type of VD from there!" This is interesting contrast. My doctors advocating heart surgery were bad doctors, but these ones were good in my thinking. Then I had to call back. I told them that "I was sorry to bother them again. I asked them how far they were from Las Vegas." She said less than fifty-five minutes. As I was planning to piggy back my pleasure trip with my next business trip, I asked them "How far from the airport?"

The word fifty-five minutes that revived my agonizing memories of going all the way to Reno to visit the other legal brothel and I had given up because it required renting a car. Her sweet voice came on again. "You do not need to rent a car, we have complimentary Limo." Would you like to me to transfer this call to Warren, he is our Limo driver! Complementary limo ride convinced me that this was a class establishment. As I was running this on my mind, she added with a sexy voice, "I can imagine what you must be thinking. Since this is your first time you wonder if this is the right place to go. Let me tell you that a lot of our clients are repeat clients. We make sure they are completely satisfied." This gave me the courage to ask the question that had meant to ask but was worried to ask.

"I am fifty-nine years old, and my wife tells me I am terrible in bed!" Then as if confessing to an old friend and confident, I added that "I have performance problem in bed. What if I could not perform?"

In a reassuring and respectful voice she said, "I understand." Then after a very short pause, she added "Remember, these ladies are professionals." Her reassuring answer prompted me to ask my next question. "Can I ask for you when I get there?" Without a hesitation she said yes. Since during the discussion she had referred to ladies and having "parties" with them as the polite word for having sex with them, I asked her "Can I party with you?"

In another nice voice, that seemed to convey a sense of sensuality and pride and respect, she said, "Please do not hesitate to ask for me. I work here from 9:00 to 5:00 six days a week. And, I will be elated to say hello to you since I am sure you are a kind and nice man. But as far as partying, I am not licensed and on top of that I am happily married. Let me take the last part back, I am for the most part happily married!" Very quickly in rapid fire she added, "However, at any given time, day or night there are twelve or so most attractive, beautiful woman in our lineup." After clearing her throat, she added that "I am about three years older than you, and I have worked here for many years as a telephone operator. So, I am not sure that you will be interested in me, as there are many "movie star" like beauties here to choose from. I liked talking to you, please ask for me, and we can have a drink together if you like."

I was a bit disappointed. I think that she sensed that and warmly asked "Do you play golf?" I said yes. "Well you can play golf here if you like. We have a nice one!"

I soon recovered from my disappointment as I looked them up in the internet. There were more than fifty world class beauties there. Between golf and these pictures, I was sold.

As a writer, I had to do my research. I went on Amazon.com and found many books about Sheri's Ranch. I ordered as many as possible and paid premium for their overnight shipment to my office. My office was much safer than home. They never opened my book packages. In contrast, if it was shipped to my home and if my wife had discovered the package she would have had a heart attack.

The package arrived the next day. I quickly opened the package.

One book talked about a nun having worked in Sheri's Ranch. A nun!

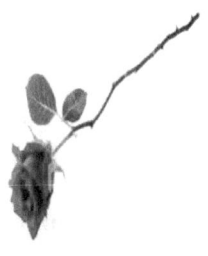

I speed read the chapter. Yes, it was true they had a former nun turned sex worker who worked there. Then there was a nurse. This nurse was astonishingly attractive; a natural blonde; beautiful breasts; long and beautiful hands; long and luring sexy legs. The unfortunate turn of events is that in her first few weeks as a nurse, a hospital employee had raped her in an empty patient room. After this she was done with nursing.

Based on the book, both of these ladies had decided that instead of hating and condemning, they would try healing their wounds and the wounds of the society. Their theory was that severe depravation and the hypocritical message of the society regarding sex is what caused these types of criminal things such as rape or even murder.

By no stretch of imagination they or I accept the criminal act of rape or other crimes of passion. Yet, they felt that serving as sex workers might help young men not to resort to stupid acts. In my case, I was a rational old man who was severely deprived and I could not take it anymore. I was not the type to have an affair. I was not the type to do anything that was illegal or unethical.

I was married and I loved my wife forever. Let me put it this way, I was married, but I was not dead.

In a visitor's guide book to Las Vegas, there was a mention of the places in Las Vegas that pretended to allow sex any time. They kept serving expensive drinks and then refused to allow any sexual activity as prostitution was illegal in Las Vegas itself.

My research had resulted in my thinking that at least on paper Sheri's Ranch was a legitimate reputable establishment. This was as far as I could tell from books.

A few weeks later, I finally picked up the phone and called Warren, the limo driver. He seemed to have a deep Brooklyn accent who told me that he would be happy to drive me from the airport to the "Ranch."

I told him that this is my first time. I asked him how much the limo ride would cost. He said it is complementary, and then he added that the ride itself is free. Then calmly he added, however a lot of clients are so happy that they give me a tip. But, this is completely optional.

I half jokingly asked him, "Do you promise not to abandon me and leave while I am inside?" I was putting the emphasis on the double intended meaning of "inside."

He had understood me perfectly well. "Sir, I am employee number fourteen and I have worked here many years. I, or any other limo drivers have never abandoned anybody inside, or outside for that matter. Come here and judge for yourself. This is a nice establishment."

Every word, by everyone I talked to was a professional, well practiced confidence builder. Nobody put pressure. There were no sales gimmicks. They all seemed to say the same thing and mean the same thing.

I had to go see this with my own eyes!

There was of course an element of risk. What if this was another of those shady places. I had gone to a topless bar many years ago in Chicago and had paid a lot of money for a date with one of the beauties there.

The date turned out to be a disappointing and complete rip off.

Excitement was building up as I was ready to visit, and have a party, with the woman of my choosing from the lineup.

I was counting the hours. I had wet dreams. I just could not wait.

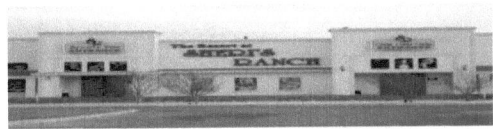

Finally after a long period of anticipation, the day arrived for my party in Sheri's Ranch.

I was ashamed, worried, excited, and horny all at the same time.

I did feel like a dirty fifty-nine year old; I also felt like a twenty year old virgin for the first time going to his honeymoon with his high school sweetheart.

The Ranch is located in a nice area with clean air. However, it is hot as it is in Nevada desert.

Warren rang the bell, and a lovely woman of around forty opened the door to greet us. She had a nice outfit and a clipboard. She took a fast glance at the clip board to double check my name and he thanked me by saying, "Mr. Condon, we thank you for your visit and your business. You are important to us!"

For a fraction of second, I thought she said, "…You are impotent…" That was my feeble mind, she had said important.

I did not have to tell them that I had anxiety. I was worried about a lot of things. Performance anxiety was the least of the anxieties.

They offered me a drink, and then without any pushing, they said please tell us when you are ready. "No rush! Please make yourself comfortable! You will be happy with us. We are here to serve you the best way possible."

When I was ready, I was escorted to another nice salon. There were several white couches, a nice coffee table with a brochure of the type of parties one could have at Sheri's Ranch in tasteful suggestive, yet accurate words. There also so was a piano in the corner.

The line up consisted of about fifteen beauties. These were like the beauties that you see in Hollywood. Some of them were in bikinis, some in lingerie, some in long night gown, and some in lather that was perhaps an indication of their specialty. None were topless, or had see through cloths, as the Ranch encouraged a fair chance for all the ladies.

Each would take a step forward and just mention their name is some sort of military precision, nothing more, and nothing less. This again was the house rule and regulations. Right after doing their introduction, they would step back right in their place in the line.

My heart beat had elevated to a level that my face was getting red. The clipboard lady came to me and whispered in my ear if I was OK, or if I had any questions.

"No questions, but I am indeed overwhelmed with all these beautiful sexy women!"

I noticed some of the ladies were standing on high heel shoes. I did not think that it was fair to them to keep them waiting, and waiting in suspense.

As if anticipating my concern, the clipboard lady assured me that I did not have to rush. I took one more look and I was sure of my decision.

I had picked Ophelia. I had seen a lot of her pictures in the Sheri's Ranch website. It was however astonishing to realize that she was taller and prettier than those pictures. She approached me and very gently took my hand to guide through a narrow hallway with big windows towards a waterfall and the golf course. But this anticipation of fun overshadowed my golf addiction urges easily.

None of the women wore any perfume. This in contrast with their counter parts in Paris. Also, there was strict code about not touching, or showing the client anything until after the fee is negotiated.

I sat down on a couch in Ophelia's room as they each have a room assigned to them when they are in the Ranch during their "Tour of Duty"

"What do like to do?" was her first question. She handed me a so called menu with sky rocketing prices. She noticed that I was not ready to pay those kinds of prices.

"We can negotiate for what you want for what you want to pay. I hope it works with me but if not there are plenty of others too."

I hate negotiations!

I mentioned in a low tone of voice a figure that even I knew was too low. To my surprise, she said that "She would be happy to stay within my budget, but there will be very little that we can party on that figure."

She explained different parties. One was "Half and Half" It consisted of oral sex, which I had never ever had in my life, and then a straight lay! Straight lay! Then as if to make my choice easier she said that I could have just the straight lay and that brings the price even lower.

Nope. I was set on the "Half and Half" treatment.

I knew in my heart of hearts that if I did not get this "Half and Half" treatment which sounded just like the half and half creamy milk you buy in any supermarket, I would regret it forever.

This regret would have been killing me since there was no guarantee that I will ever come back there as this was expensive and frankly, I did not really know if it was going to be a good experience.

She added another $100 to my "Half and Half" offer and she said that I need to pay first. I did, as I could not wait to see how glamorous this beauty looked in her birthday suit.

My eyes popped out when I saw her in the nude.

Her body was perfect. Her face was perfect. She was by far the most beautiful woman I had ever seen in Europe, or here.

The house rule mandated condoms at all times.

She put a condom on me patiently but professionally. Then she tested it to make sure it was in place. I felt I was having a fever. There was just too much visual excitation and she had not touched me yet.

"Honey, do like the oral first?"

I looked down and I could not believe my own eyes! I was as hard as a rock. My answer, as if she could not see my erect penis, was that I was fully ready. Let us for oral first. "Do you prefer soft, or with a bit more pressure?"

I was doing the best I could to stay alert. "Would you like to lie down? I can do it any shape or form you like." As if talking to a trusted lover of many years, I only had to shyly mention that this was my first time ever. I had never had oral sex. I told her that I was not even sure that I will like it. She gave me a convincing response by saying "You will like it. And if you do not, we will do something else instead. Our goal is to completely satisfy you."

Aside from her lips gently brushing against the upper side of my penis, I could not feel anything with the portion that was in the condom. "You cannot feel anything." She had sensed it and she was right. "In that case, I will use a different kind of condom which is the sensitive type."

Jackpot! That was the brand I used when I was single and twenty-five years younger. How could she have guessed? She suggested that it might be a good idea for me to sit right next to her as she carefully put the sensitive condoms on me. They were the lubricated type and the more expensive type that I had always used and trusted.

She unrolled the condom and put it on. She did this effortlessly with all her charm and stunning beauty. My most erotic movie screen dream was being acted not in dream land but in reality. "Man you are beautiful, clean and thick!" This boosted my confidence and removed all doubts about the performance anxiety. Then as if that was not enough, she asked, "Did you notice that I had to completely unroll the condom?" Since this was a rhetorical question, I hesitated to answer.

"You are bigger than about 80% of the general white population. You are also very white and clean." I was elated to hear these things. Nobody had ever told me these. I had heard bits and pieces, but never in such a confident, assuring, and sexy way. All my inhibitions flew out the window.

She knew exactly what to do and say when and how in the most exquisite sensual way. It was not just sex. It was most fulfilling sex art.

Then she said, "OK, you are ready for the other half!" It did seem, and actually was the case that this was the case. Even I was impressed by my own performance in the hands of this glamorous Venus.

The other half was not just as effortless as the first half. I needed to do some of the "work" as well. She noticed. "Honey do you want something else?" I said, "I know that I had not negotiated this in advance, but, may I kiss you?"

The answer to this is usually no in Europe. Some sex workers leave the kisses on their lips for their husbands. This is a private and dignified way to keep a distinction between work sex and love sex reserved for their loved ones.

I had always, always honored this, but without kiss, I would not be able to "perform well." It seemed like we had reached a dead end. Voices in my head told me, "See this is where she is going to jack up the price! I told you so! Here you are! You are not as smart as you think!"

"I see. We did not negotiate this. But you can kiss anywhere you like!"

The party was back on! Like a school boy who was kissing for the first time ever, and getting all the pleasure related to that, I was in heaven.

The second kiss was all I needed to enter her.

The straight lay was the best I had ever had.

Once it was all over, she got back on the bed and slept right next to me and hugged me. Her cupped hands were carefully holding my penis and testicles. They are extremely careful about seaman. They do not want it spill or they are very careful about any bodily liquid exchange. Bodily liquid exchange is the source of AIDS and they know what to do. Her cupped long fingers, although a powerful source of excitement, were a calculated exercise in being in control of my seaman and making sure that it will not spill.

She asked, "Do you want to go for some more?" The answer was, and always will be "yes, yes, and yes!"

While it was true that I had "performed well" far way above and beyond my expectations or imaginations there was no guarantee if I could be able to receive or absorb any more.

She put her panties on and the long dress, and asked if she could go get some cold drink.

She came back with a nice ice basket containing several bottles of water. The water was chilled. A powerful taste quencher considering that the temperature outside this comfortably air conditioned room would reach 114 degrees that day.

"I think that you will enjoy a nice carry." "Can you carry me to the door?" I am not too experienced, but I was able to follow what she was saying. Standing up as I was, she wanted for me to enter her and be face to face while walking, as is I was carrying her across the room."

"This was another thing that I had never ever done before!" It worked its intended charm, pleasure, and delight!

I was completely satisfied the way I was never satisfied before. I kept looking at their website once or twice a day.

One day there was a headline about Air Force Amy. She had represented Sheri's Ranch in the regional competition. I had worked overtime and extremely hard and I felt that I deserved this. The picture angle was such that I could easily guess how her beautiful breast must look like without the bra. I longed for that.

I called and set up an appointment with Air Force Amy.

From then on it looked as if Warren would be my designated driver each and every time and I was happy with this arrangement. We always talked like we were good old friends while driving to and away from the Ranch.

I was not too surprised to find out that each lady was an independent contractor and they set their own fees and their own partying rules.

Negotiation was swift and I was giving this nude lady a hug soon. Her breasts were touching my chest in the most delightful way imaginable. This time however, I was smart to have had negotiated kissing in advance. I started by kissing her breasts.

Then I was sort of urging her to sit on top of me. She knew what brand of condom to use, and she was ready for action. She was sitting on top in the most natural way right after a short period of sensual massage to my penis.

My penetration was deep and extremely enjoyable.

"Does this feel good to you?" Then in a very sexy voice she added, "This feels very sexy to me!" Then she squished me inside, made a side by side move with me almost sobbing, "Do this, I like this, it feels great!" Her answer was "OK" then "I will do whatever pleases you!"

I looked across the room and noticed my clothes on the sofa. There was my shirt and pants. Then what turned me on even more, was her beautiful white satin panties that were placed on top on my pants. Her panties were nicely folded, clean and white and soft and right next to the zipper on my pants.

"If you stay hard, you can relieve yourself as long as condom stays on!" My prayers were answered the condom staid on, and I came.

It seemed that this was the only entertainment I needed in my life. It had been months and months after I had any sex with my wife and even then I had a sense that I was pushing her to do what she really did not like to do. As a result of menopause, she had absolutely no desire for sex. No desire at all.

What was I supposed to do? After all I was a man. I was a man who could have easily ended up on wheelchair after the spine surgery.

Sex deprivation was getting me go out of my mind.

One day in Crispy Cream donuts shop, I got excited about jelly filled glazed donuts. They did look like a breast. The jelly inside that was visible from outside, did indeed look like a nipple that had lipstick on it. This is a turn on for many men.

The chocolate glazed plain donuts, reminded me of kissing a beautiful woman who had a chocolate colored lipstick. This was another turn on for me. As if to put salt on my sexual depravation wound, there was "Half and Half" cream near the coffee.

This was it. I picked the phone and called the Ranch. I made a reservation with Kat.

Kat's picture on the website shows a most attractive woman with professional make up. She looks somewhat like Joan Rivers. Her cleavage and her big breasts suggest an exquisite level of sensuality and sexual pleasure.

On the way there, Warren had to call several times to tell them where we were on our way and an estimate of our arrival time. This was for two reasons. I had told Warren on the phone that I was taking Viagra. Viagra works only within a certain time frame, beyond that it is ineffective. So, Warren was well aware of the time frame and made sure that we arrive there in the right time.

The second reason was that Kat was having a party with another client that day right before me. The anticipation of going to bed with one of the most beautiful and sexy women in the world added to excitement. I could not wait. However, I knew well that the waiting with the added excitement will make the climax peak even higher and deeper!

Kat is a drop dead beauty. She drinks only coffee and she likes to chew sugarless gums.

She works by the hour and she is proud of her superb work. In most pictures she is wearing an elegant but unpretentious watch. I read this to say that she goes by the hour.

Kat is from Los Angeles, and her kisses are the best. Her kisses and kisses alone made me come before there was any other sexual activity. Her lips are the shapeliest lips I have ever seen.

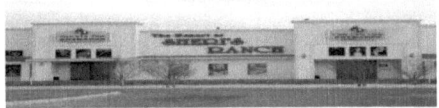

CHAPTER 18:
Angelina

As totally satisfied as I was from my previous partying with Kat, I heard from another executive that "Bryce, you need to check out Angelina. She is fire!"

Just like an alcoholic, I thought that I had my last drink with partying with Kat. In particular Kat had a strong resemblance to Roya. So, I had gotten my fill. I was satisfied.

These things are not that inexpensive.

OK, I ignored the urges at first. Then I felt that I had to check this out even though I had been fulfilled before. I had sex with one of the most attractive women on earth namely, Kat. As if it was OK, I had closed my eyes and imagined that Kat was Roya that I did not have a chance to make love too.

I had felt that sex with Kat, had been from the universe making amends to me. This amend was for not have been given a chance to make love to Roya.

The fact that Roya was twenty-some years prior to this did not even make any difference. I was hurt and I was hurt bad in that process.

I was sitting in front of my computer waiting for my next flight at Orlando Airport in Florida. I was bored and I missed my wife and children a great deal. Somehow as if it was not under my control, I ended up at the website that showed Angelina.

Oh, my God!

Angelina looked just like that sexpot girl that was in "Married with Children." Just the thought of her beauty and sexiness would make me hot.

For three days, I just could not get her out of my mind. I tried and tried as hard as I could. Unfortunately nothing worked. Knowing that she was just a telephone call away, added to the burden.

Right about then, the Computer Electronics Show being held in Las Vegas. I and three others were asked to go to this show and represent our company. I arrived in Las Vegas and had a drink and went directly to the show.

At the entrance, there was a sexy woman in hot pants registering seminar goers.

I quickly did the registration trying to avoid temptation by not even looking at those shapely legs.

A few isles away, there was a stunningly beautiful sex goddess who was doing a show on our competition's company products. The main reason for us being there was to see what the competition was saying.

All three of us were sitting in the front row wishing that the competition somehow would not see our company logo on our name tag. The show was short and the CEO of the completion came and shook our hands and did something we did not really anticipate.

He took me on the side and said, "Bryce, go tell that empty headed CEO of your company that I want to sign a contract that will bring our companies $2.3 Million in one year. We can split that in half. Tell that idiot to stop playing games with us. This will be good for both of us!" The other two tried to get into this confidential discussion, but no luck for them. "Here, you give this contract to him and him alone! Nobody else needs to see this. If I hear that anyone else has heard about this, I will see to it that you get fired!" Then, there came a backhanded compliment. "Bryce you are damn good. You are so good that we hate you. But keep in mind that both our companies have failed in getting this contact acting alone. You are an old man, you know what I say. Go kick this guy into reality." Before I could even open my mouth, he pushed the contact in my face. Then with a smile on his face, he said that he personally wanted to invite me to his company's hospitality room at Flamingo. "There are two girls for each guy. Food is prepared by an executive chef from Maxim of Paris! Oh, you need the password to get in. The password is Barry White. Do not bring the others as this is a single invitation."

Barry White for God's sake is the guy who sang "Sexual Healing" song in a very deep masculine voice.

If I was going to bring in $2.3 Million contract, as it seemed like this contract would be, I deserved a little break.

I had to have Angelina!

I called warren first. "Where are you? It has been over a year since you had a little party here. What is going on? You do not like us anymore?" I had to disrupt him. "Hey Warren, I am here in Vegas. Can you get an appointment with Angelina for me?" The answer was a terse "Call you back!" This was with the typical efficiency that they have.

My cell phone rang in less than a minute. "But you have to be there in less than two hours. She has an appointment in four hours from now! Can you do it?" He said, "What a question to ask. I will make sure that I will make it."

I hopped into Warren's Limo and we were on our way to the Ranch. Warren knew many of my life's secrets, heart breaks, hopes, and problems. I am positive that either he made mental notes or he would write things down somewhere about each client.

As always he was really interested in being a friend. As we were approaching the Ranch, he made just one comment. He said "Bryce, Angelina is not cheap but she is worth every penny!" Then with a friendly smile we shook hands and I was greeted by Angelia.

Angelina escorted me to her room. Her room was a bit bigger than other rooms. She had short blonde hair. Her hair was shiny just like new minted gold. Her body was absolutely perfect.

She sat next to me on the couch and asked "What is on your mind, and how can you please you today?" Our negotiations were more involved that before. Fortunately, we arrived at a conclusion.

In her bio at the Ranch website, I had read that she liked to shop at Victoria's Secret. Later on, she had written that this, meaning working at the Ranch, has been her life dream. It also added that she is having a lot of fun in Las Vegas.

She was hotter than I was. She was not going to waste any time. Her kisses made me go up in flames. Since premature ejaculation had been my worry before, she asked if she could be in charge of timing. After all she was the professional. Straight Lay, oral sex, breast massage, were all expertly inter twined. The sensation was just out of this world. I had never ever had been so excited. I was so excited that I was shivering. She was riding me when I had to utter the word "Now, now!" This was asking her to help me come. Like an experienced cowboy riding on a horse, she shifted her weight so ever slightly. This gave arousal to parts of my penis that I knew will bring me to a climax. Then seconds later, she moved up a bit, and sat back on me again.

This last in and out motion had made me come right after she said "Now!" I exploded with a big sigh of relief. She was beginning to repeat the upward motion when I begged her not to move. I was so sensitive that any slight motion would have been beyond my human pleasure capacity.

Then as she was still sitting on top of me, she said, "Man, you are strong, hard, thick, and you have an excellent plunger action" I did hear all of these, but they did not register. I did mean to ask her what plunger action meant but I forgot. I was too excited! I truly felt like a fourteen year old virgin experiencing climax for the first time ever!

As she escorted me back to the salon as they always did, she whispered in my ear that she will be there another two weeks. "Come back for a butterfly next time!" she said as she kissed me again, and gave me a big and sensual hug.

I had been told that I was not good in bed before. Nevertheless, my sex education never consisted of knowing about butterflies or plunger action!

Now, I had to find out these new terms meant! I knew that I just had to!

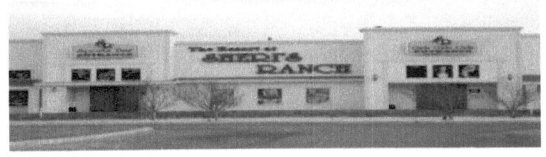

Chapter 19:
Gabriella

I Picked Gabriella from the second line up I ever had in my life at the Ranch.

She looked and behaved just like a young and sexy college professor even though she was in her thirties. Her hair was colored a sparkling silver and it was sassy. Unlike Kat and Angelina, her breasts were smaller but enticingly shapely. The amazing thing was that they bounced around like jelly. I noticed that her shoes were low heel shoes. Still, she was six feet tall with amazingly beautiful legs.

Her legs reminded me of a Pan American Airlines' flight attendant legs that I loved for a while. This beautiful Swedish natural blonde, has such beautiful legs that a book was written about them. Indeed, those legs were so shapely that she ended up becoming a Hollywood star. Part of this was because her legs looked like Marylyn Monroe.

"Bryce, tell me, Are you a university professor?"

"No, but I wished I was!"

"Are you?"

"Not really. But I do have a Master's degree in Psychology!"

I could see that Gabriella was different from others at the Ranch. She was first trying to talk to me before there were any negotiations or the slightest physical touch. Suddenly, I started to worry. I worried because in one of the first negotiation seminars I ever had as a manager, we were taught to really understand your opponent. Try to figure out what made him or her tick. "Aha, this is what she is trying to do! She is doing this to jack up the prices!" I told myself.

The truth was that she really wanted to carry an intelligent conversation about all those years that she worked on her Master's degree. She also was trying to find out how best to please me. This I figured out for certain when she said she did not like negotiations either; she told me that she is lover first and a business person second; she told me that some things are more important than money in this world.

Then in passing she said thanks to me for selecting her and making her entertain my sexual, intellectual, and sentimental thoughts. Then she added, "Ranch rules state that we need to negotiate a fee for whatever activity that you have in mind."

Before, I could answer her, my cell phone rang. My smart phone was programmed to ring in a special way when something urgent needed attention at work. This was that ring tone that I learned to hate and at the worst possible time.

"What is the emergency?" I asked in a cold and calculated voice. It was one of the colleagues from the company who had accompanied me to the Consumer Electronics Show in Las Vegas. In an urgent voice muffled by the fact that he must have held his hand around his phone so others cannot hear, he pleaded with me. "Bryce, we are in Flamingo and our competition is having a hospitality suite. You cannot believe the number of super attractive women who are here. Our competition always beat us hands down in these things. Man, this is super target rich zone!"

Then in a totally disappointing voice he added "Some of these women are so sexy that I have wetted my pants. Please, please, please tell us the password since without that we cannot sneak in!" Then as if I had not heard it the first time, with a moaning sound close to crying and like a four year old who has fallen in love with a toy, he added "Please, please, please!"

I always hated it when a grown man cried.

"Barry White!"

His startled sound, again in a muffled tone asked to confirm, "Barry White? Barry White? Hell my wife gets turned on by his voice and that is precisely the reason I hate his guts! I be damned, Barry White!" The last uttering of Barry White was good enough for the bouncer to allow them both in.

It must have, otherwise the phone would have not gone silent. After I hung up, Gabriella asked, "Barry White? Do you like him? I have some of his music!" "No, no, I hate his voice. I admit that he is an excellent singer that my wife and my colleague go crazy for. This is why I do not like him, or actually his voice!" "I understand! This is male jealousy, or envy?"

"Let us continue the negotiations." In an aloof voice, as if she was above it all, she said, "I know you are a repeat customer. Tell me what you paid for the same services the last times you were here, and I will make you a deal!" I mentioned the figure. She stood right near me, kissed me in the ear and said, "OK, but I will give you a 15% discount for the intellectual conversation we just had. We are all independent contractors here and we set our own fees!" She was smart, because she had accurately figured out the exact amount.

As she left to give the money to the cashier, again according to the Ranch rules, I remembered something very sweet that I had heard from her. She had told me that sex meant a lot between our ears that it really meant between our legs. "Surprisingly enough, our most important pleasure center is our brain and not what we think it is!"

Our partying started rapidly. It somehow felt like she was hungrier for sex than I was. Of course, being professionals, they do know what the right speed and extend of the partying is for each client and they respect that.

If indeed it was true that the sex act has a lot more with the brain than with our manhood, this psychological experiment had established proof of it.

"Relax, let go of the past. Enjoy the moment!" She said this in a commanding, yet convincing, and caring way. At that point, we had consumed the "Straight lay" portion of our contract. As if to catch her breath and to rejoice in the pleasure, she asked if she can go get a drink. "Sure" was my answer. This will let me cool down and relax for the second half of the main event.

In a few seconds, she had put on her night dress, and left the room without any panties underneath. She reappeared just as quickly as she had left with two glasses of Cognac in her hands. "Bryce, for your superb performance, you deserve this! It is on me!" I could not really believe what was happening. I thanked her and had a sip.

Her cognac glass had smudges of her chocolate tinted soft purple colored lipstick. I could clearly see that since her glass was almost empty. She then carefully put both glasses on the dresser nearby and sat right next to me.

Her leg was gently touching my leg reminding me of my third grade love! Gabriella's shaved long beautiful legs made my hairy legs look ugly and undesirable. But somehow she was not looking at my legs. She was absorbed into thinking of something a lot deeper than the pleasures of the moment. I will never know what she was thinking about.

She then resumed the "activities" with a zeal combined with such elegance and romance that only a famous Hollywood actress of big fame can deliver on the screen.

I was shivering. I felt for a long second as if my heart had stopped. I was breathing normally, but it felt like my entire being was consumed in a sweet way with the best that nature could offer! It indeed was sweet surrender of my entire being to this lovely and loving creature.

She was not having sex with me. She was making love to me and I to her in that party!

I was too excited to perform. I was cursing myself. She effortlessly realized what is going on. She in that soft commanding voice asked me to put my head on her shoulder for a minute and relax. Then she moved so ever slightly so my head was gently placed between her vacillating breasts. She placed one hand over my head and sang a lullaby song for me. It felt I was hallucinating. But I was not!

I started to feel hard as rock again. When her hand touched me, I got even stronger. She then said "Let us go back to where we left out! Ready!"

After we were done, I realized one gigantic deep sexual and emotional satisfaction that was indeed super natural. At least for those precious moments of climax, my "Blonde Blues" were poetically morphed into a super sensation of experiencing an erupting volcano of intense and immense pleasure. The "Blonde Blue" mirage of sex being one and only thing, brain washed into my psyche for all these years, was being felt by my entire shivering being as if they were the entire reason d'être of my being.

I was magically and holistically had been transformed for those "forever" few peak heavenly delicious instants! Instants that I had longed for millenniums it seemed.

There is a lingerie shop right in the departure lounge of McCarran Airport in Las Vegas. This shop has a tasteful collection of panties as well. I overcame my shyness and ventured inside. An elegant looking saleswoman slowly made eye contact and then approached me without any pressure. "Are you interested in bikinis, briefs, or honeymoon specialty panties?" As the word panties was coming out of her beautiful lips and while I was noticing here model level cleavage sexily put on display, I was desperately longing for sex again. Right at that moment, my silent self-talk went off life a fire cracker. "Bryce, really, you just had sex less than an hour ago! You were satisfied, less than an hour ago! Now you want more? Do you really want more sex? Man, you must be out of your mind? I know do not tell me, you want sex with this one! Is that right? Use your real brain, not the one that you usually use which is between your legs!"

When I finished my check-in for the next leg of my trip and sat down, my mind again raced back to my party with Gabriella.

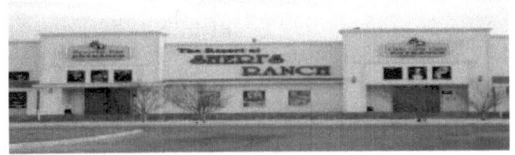 CHAPTER 20:
Sheri's Ranch
Line Ups

Theoretically at Sheri's Ranch, any time of day or night a visitor can ask for a line up, and there will be some ten to fifteen of the most beautiful sexy women who would line up. On the occasions that I have been there, I have found this to be a powerful way to get me ready for action, or actually super action. This is especially true since visually seeing these alluring sexy women completes what Viagra cannot do alone. While it is impossible to tell if one of these irresistible ladies would be a more satisfying partner than the others for an individual, there is always the negotiation stage. During that time, a particular sexual activity or the other can be discussed and then one can find out if the person was chosen from the lineup will be the right partner.

On one of my few visits there, I saw a tall and athletic man carefully review the lineup. Then he decided on one particular lady. They disappeared through the hall way going to her room. Then, much to my surprise, they returned in a few minutes.

The man waited in the bar for about ten minutes, and then another lady came out and they went to her room. This time, they did not return quickly.

The bar tender, noticing my surprise, explained what might have happened. She said that "During the negotiations they must have figured out they were not as suitable for each other as they first thought. So, the first lady recommended another one that was more suitable. The second lady who showed up in the bar was sent by the first one." Then she went on, "This happens not very often, but it does happen. The ladies are very nice about this. By introducing another lady, they keep the customer happy. Also, who knows, the same courtesy will be extended to them later on."

On my second visit, while I was choosing from the lineup, I noticed that a few locals were sitting in the bar as if they were observing and carefully immersed in watching a beauty contest. They were astonished by the number of beauties that were on the lineup.

This is the ultimate of the ultimate!

Ultimate is that so many times in the movies or parties, we find some attractive woman. However, men being what they are, we tell ourselves, I wish she was taller, or she was a bit more top-heavy, whatever else.

Nevertheless, in a lineup situation, you find women of all kinds. That gave me the ultimate that I was looking for.

I do not want to say that all of my visits were perfect. On my third visit, I had carefully picked one of the most gorgeous women. She gently offered to hold my hand as we strolled in a long hallway that is between the big living room where line ups happen and that individual lady's room. They usually walk elegantly on their high heel shoes.

Upon arriving in her room, I noticed that she looked totally exhausted. As we started to discuss what I had in mind for our "party" she seemed to look down a bit and then try to keep a smile as well as the eye to eye contact.

"Honey, what you are asking for is quite reasonable. I would have normally been extremely happy to give you this pleasure. However, I am running out of energy. However, we could still do it if you want. Nevertheless, I think that Heidi might be a better partner for you today." Then with a bigger smile than what she had managed to produce before, she asked if it was OK for her to take me to Heidi's room.

On the way back Warren explained what had happened. They had a marathon, mega party the day and night before. A club had reserved the entire Ranch. "Almost all ladies were busy most of the time. Some even had two or three guys waiting for them to finish one party before they went to the next. So, I think right now some of them must be a bit exhausted." I understood that. He then went on to say that he himself had had to drive this route three times during the last twenty-four hours. In spite all of this, he looked dapper as usual. Then with that thick Brooklyn he added "Good thing is that I usually manage to take a nap here and there and a good clean shower and shave while clients are in there." It seemed like there was no pun intended in the "in there" phrase.

I have often wondered what he meant by "while they were in there". Did he mean when the clients' lipstick was actually in the ladies' lipstick case? Or, he innocently just was referring to while the clients were in the ladies room. The "in there" part is erotically confusing.

Being a man, and after all that expensive partying, I still had to do a woman called "Air Force Ami". She seemed to show up once in a while. Her DD-sized beautifully sculptured breasts have been a longing heated desire of mine for a long time. Unfortunately, my schedule and hers were always in direct conflict. This goes to prove that if a man was able to party with all the women in the Ranch except for one, he will have burning longing for "the one that got away" even though he had had great sex with all the rest. This is the man conditioning that men are wired with for centuries. I continue to feel the heat for Air Force Amy!

One of the books about this Ranch talked about what kind of man goes there. It referred to David. David was a handsome man. He was presentable, and he did not have any particular problem finding women.

So the question is why he was a repeat customer here. The answer was that he wanted a safe to have sex with a beautiful woman and then not get involved.

This was a clean cut way for him to get the satisfaction that he would not get unless he was involved. With my little knowledge of psychology, I think that women get involved with sex to build relationships, and men the other way around.

Going back to Gabriella putting my head on her chest and her singing me a lullaby song, she was doing what she knew best as woman. She was making intimacy and relationship.

Even though this intimacy was just for temporary and for an hour or two, it was what she instinctively knew best.

"I am ready when you are ready. There is no rush. Here put your head on my shoulder!"

I felt like I was young again. I was emotionally transported to the best of times of my youth; the immense land of nostalgia; the intense emotions of happiness. Even though the "good old days" were never really as good as we now think they were. Of course at my age, some of my body parts were not as agile as they used to be when I was twenty, or thirty. Astonishingly enough, with a partner like this, one regains the youth.

The youth and related manhood, are also just as temporary as Gabriella had kept alive with her intimacy effort. For that moment, I felt young with a strong feeling of manhood. This was thanks to Gabriella for fueling my sexual desire and managing to keep it alive and functional.

On those moments that my head was on her shoulder, I remembered my marriage.

My wife is totally different from Gabriella. But, I remember that I used to get same feelings when I placed my head on her shoulder. I felt secure, happy, while I cared for them. This is a genuine emotion that last a few seconds and is bolstered for those moments with the feeling of contentment.

In fact in my old age I am arrived at a conclusion that all women are pretty. All women are like Mona Lisa! They try to make a nest. They try to make a home.

I had noticed that Gabriella would make sure that our drinks are on coasters. She did not want to damage the furniture. My wife was the same. She had carefully selected our chinaware and really took good care of them. The fact was that we had bought the plates in a big sale. They were not elegant or stylish, but they were the glue that kept our home going. Suddenly a perfect storm rocked my entire existence as I was sitting next to Gabriella and thinking those thoughts. "Bryce, how dare you to sit here and even think about your wife?" Feeling intense guilt and shame, I could not answer that question right at that moment in time.

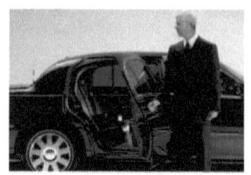 CHAPTER 21: Warren, My Confidant and Limousine Driver

The limo driver, who picked me up from my house in Chicago, was from the limo company that had a contract with the company that I worked for. They seem to send a different driver each time and most of them did not say much except for "Good Morning Mr. Condon. Even at saying this, sometimes there would be an embarrassing moment when they had to look up my name from a computer print out. "Are you going to O'Hare Airport today? Are you on United Airlines flight 958 to London, Heathrow?"

As if I was insulted, or if somebody had intentionally had put salt on my wound, I sneered at the driver "No, No, No!" I am going to Las Vegas on United 980 which departs at 8:26!" I got really mad at this incompetent driver for trying to destroy my elaborate plans for having sex with some of the most attractive women in the world. I even thought that this was part of conspiracy to deny me my last chance at sex after what seemed centuries of deprivations.

That would have been really awful!

The internist had told me that the cardiologist had ordered all those angiograms, and stress tests and other things because he was suspecting that I had an enlarged heart. Then as if trying to endear himself to me at the expense of the cardiologist, he shifted in his chair but quickly sat back. I never liked this guy. Now, my disgust and distrust of him had even grown further. I knew that he had something he wanted to tell me, but was holding back.

"Doctor, please tell me what you were about to say" I emphatically told him.

Just like a defendant that would take the fifth amendment in a hostile trial, he pulled back even further. Suddenly, as if feeling sorry for me, he started in his mono tone voice again.

He said "With your health risks, your medical history, especially the heart attack at an early age, we think that you do have an enlarged heart, an enlarged heart just like your father had at much later stage of his life. Nevertheless, we need these tests to tell you this."

It felt like a criminal was trying to forge evidence for a crime that he was planning to do. Were they trying to kill me?

It took me a few minutes to get my exposure back. "Doctor, suppose the tests say I have an enlarged heart. If so, how long would I have to live?"

I could see a twinkle in his eyes as if he had just conquered highest peaks on Alps! Then he started to talk. This time he was preaching with authority and confidence. "Well, generally life expectancy in such cases is measured in quarters."

After feeling like being shucked by a million volts of electricity, I had no problem figuring out what he meant. Each quarter in calendar is three months. So, he was telling me that I had at least three months or as much as nine months or a year to live!

"Damn you doctor! You are not God, the hell with you, doctor. You do not know what the hell you are talking about!" I am glad that I just thought these thoughts, but did not verbalize them.

I started to think ahead about my fun trip to Las Vegas!

It had snowed all the night before and it was cold and usual Chicago wind howling, as we drove to the airport listening to classical music in the limo's outstanding sound system. The limo company had made a notation in my profile that I loved classical music. So, the driver quickly switched to my station as I sat inside. He had been listening to all sports radio station that was his favorite.

I had been to Las Vegas airport many times before. Sadly, I had never been there for fun. It was always for some convention or the other. This time was different. I was going to rejuvenate, regroup, and revive myself with sex with the best of the best!

A few steps outside the terminal, Warren was waiting for me right outside a stretched limo. A big smile and a firm handshake from him reminded me of other business trips where I met other senior managers with a similar handshake. His smile and warmth was in total contrast with the one who had picked me up in Chicago.

"We are delighted that you decided to come. Trust me, you will not be disappointed." He then offered me a cold drink from quite a big selection in the car.

As we were driving, I thought that Warren must have it made. He can have sex with the most beautiful women any time he wants. After all, it must be free, or next to nothing for him. He probably gets them at employee rate.

I noticed that he could see me in his rear view mirror. I wondered if he could also hear my thoughts as my wife could. Luckily he did not have that capability.

"Mr. Condon, may I ask if this is your first time?" His second question and comment came right after the first. "If I am not wrong, this must be your first time!" My response was "Guilty as charged! I am a virgin!"

He asked me if I preferred to listen to music or watch TV. Then he added that if I had some questions, he would be more than happy to answer. Then, "Let me assure you, you will be happy with us today!"

Warren seemed to be a few years older than me. He was what I classify as a conversationalist. He was so good in carrying a conversation that he could have made a superb radio talk show host in any major city. So, I told him this. His immediate reaction was, "No. I will not enjoy the stress and the fame. This is what I can do, and I am happy with this."

The last portion of his answer was what I badly needed to hear before I asked my next question. I asked, "How are the fringe benefits?" He politely explained they are same as everywhere else; medical and dental insurance is covered; two weeks of vacation each year, and etc."

"No, I meant fringe benefits as far as all these sexy women were concerned!" He replied "No sir, just like any other reputable business, we cannot even touch the merchandize! It is strictly forbidden for us to party with the ladies. We will lose our jobs!" His answer was difficult for me to believe.

I told him he was too relaxed and seemed totally satisfied as I was when I was single and had multiple girl friends in the height of the sexual revolution. Then I asked for an apology right after that for having asked something inappropriate.

"No Mr. Condon, there is absolutely no need to apologize." The company has treated me well all these years. That is why I appear happy. However, like you I am also married and I have one child. The company, especially a company like this, cannot survive if they do not meet strict rules and regulations. No exceptions. No drugs. No partying with ladies. I cannot even come here as a guest for as long as I work here." "No sir, we are professionals. This is a good job and I do not want to lose it especially after all these years!"

Being a first timer I asked him about how things worked there and asked for advice.

He was sincere and answered my questions to the best of his ability. This was similar to a manager from one company asking a manager form other company. It is granted that they cannot give out company confidential information, but they usually say what they can say in a straight way.

Warren talked and acted just like any other professional Director or VP would talk to his or her counterparts from other company asking similar questions.

The trip from the Las Vegas Airport to Sheri's Ranch passes through high altitude mountains that have snow in the winter. There also is striking views of the mountains in the low levels on the other parts of the trip. This trip on and itself is a great sightseeing.

On one occasion, I even invited Warren to lunch. He expressed his great gratitude. However, that would have also been against company rules and regulations.

During the second visit, I had requested to talk to the Madam for a few minutes. I was not even sure that they had a Madam. They did.

The Madam was a business woman who was aware of everything that was going on there. She too told me that sometimes, it is the thrill of chase. Sometimes it is having what we cannot have that brings people here. In addition she pointed out that Sheri's Ranch is a classy and respected place with many repeat clients. She did not say customers, she said clients!

I was about to tell her my entire medical history and my disgust for having only "quarters" to live. Somehow, I was lucky. She started to share something with me. She said "Life is precious and sweat. Best things to enjoy in life and beauty are so abundant in this short life." Indeed, it is a "Short life". I wondered if she knew about me.

Warren waiting to take me back to the airport. This was such a monumental thing in my life that I started to completely trust Warren.

I felt like I was flying in could nine. I felt just as young as when I had had saturation sex in Amsterdam Red Light District. The fact remains that when I went to Amsterdam I was twenty-seven. The ride back to the airport was extremely pleasant.

Warren told me about his trip to Europe when he was twenty-five for his honeymoon. He seemed to be a world class traveler from what he told me. We talked about taking the Euro Rail train excursions that saved a lot of money. We talked about our marriages. We talked about Democrats and Republicans. He was well informed about everything.

As we approached the airport departures, I noticed that he was slowing in down near a domestic United Airlines stop. I quickly reminded him that I was flying to London. That should depart from the International Terminal.

Without hesitating for a second, or looking up any list, he said "You are on United 309. Is that right?" I said yes. "OK sir, then, for this United flight that leaves at 3:40 PM, you will be flying to San Francisco first. Then there is stopover of about one hour and twenty minutes, and then you will catch the San Francisco to London, Heathrow flight."

When people say London Heathrow, as opposed to London airport, I can tell that they have travelled enough. They have travelled enough to know that major cities have multiple airports and we need to be specific.

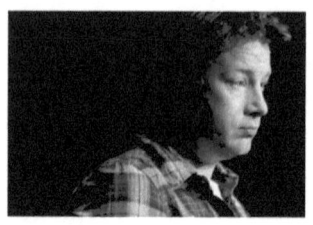

CHAPTER 22: My Last Loves For Ever

I was daydreaming about my wife, Roya, or Gabriella when suddenly I realized that this is almost the end of escape and soon I will have to be under the care of a doctor and perhaps even in a hospital.

The thought, made me disgusted and super nervous.

I had just rebelled against my own reality in a fantasy world; I had just had saturation sex roughly same levels as my younger days; I was feeling rejuvenated; I had just experienced the sexual healing that was in songs; I had just gone through what I thought sex therapy was supposed to be, and now I had to wake up! I had to wake up to cold and unfair life that had made me angry in the first place.

My wife, "claiming that she had wasted many years of life with me!" was waiting for me to get home. My brother had invited me to an excellent opera. My sister was going to take me out to dinner to "Show Off her platinum credit card, and buy me dinner!"

My bank had just leveled sky rocketing interests on my credit card and the CEO of one of the places that I worked for was being accused for incompetence as a CEO!

If there is a poetic justice, this was it! I had my last tango in Las Vegas. I had revived my limitless human power not to be a medical diagnosis or a victim. As far as I could tell I was just as good as when I was thirty.

More importantly, now I was free.

I had given the freedom to myself to be alive.

Mama Cass has a song about being free when you have nothing to lose. In addition I had rediscovered my own gutsy self. This is the same gutsy self that I had put on mute all these years. This is also the same gutsy voice that I had chocked in myself all these years.

Sitting right next to one of the sexiest, elegant, European, well educated therapist, I had chosen to be too shy to bring up these wounds. I had learned to bury them so deep that it took years before this outstanding therapist could help me cope and heal.

Do not get me wrong. Being a professional my therapist would never recommend for me to visit sex workers.

However, she helped me bring these wounds to my recent memory and then try to cope. One of the songs that have had a great impact on me for many years is "The House of the Rising Sun." The song which is about a brothel in Saint Luis says that many a young men were devastated by it. It also has a touching lyric such as "Tell your young children; not to do what I have done …"

Well, this time I was not young, therefore I was exempt from this advice.

I got another bill from my doctors that will break the bank again. This bill hit me between the eyes the same way that some cold water will bring a drunk back to being sober.

Doctors, Hospitals, Banks, CEOs, and "Bring it on!" I am Free! The love of all these women in my splurge and the sex has made me free and alive. I am no longer bounded by the no win predicament nailed to my soul that I had only "Quarters" to live.

The only quarters, I could remember were not this death sentence of having only quarters to live. The quarters I remember is the quarter drink we used to have in college. We would fill up a glass with beer. Then, we were to bounce a quarter on the table. If that quarter landed in the drink glass, then you could drink it. Otherwise, the next player would take the chance with his/her quarter. This game was affectionately known as the quarter drink.

I also strongly believe in the saying that it is better to have loved and then lost, rather than have never had loved. I will always love Roya as that love that was lost quickly. I nevertheless love her forever. Whatever Roya was and now is in my dreams, my wife is the "earth angle" realistic example of that love. Especially after our children were born, my love for my wife is eternal.

I also have learned that loving someone does not mean liking everything they were or did. In fact if I have learned anything about love is that it helps us overlook what we do not like in our loves.

Maybe, I would have had a better life with either Roya or Gabriella had I had married them. However, the famous here and now of my life is that I have married the woman that I have married. I am not stupid enough to try to change the history.

If I was to die today, I would definitely be able to say, "It was a nice life!" and go quietly and peacefully. Unlike my father before me, I cannot think of anything at this moment in time that I want to do and I had not done. I gracefully accept that my time like anybody else on this earth is limited.

CHAPTER 23: Hugh Grant and Tiger Woods

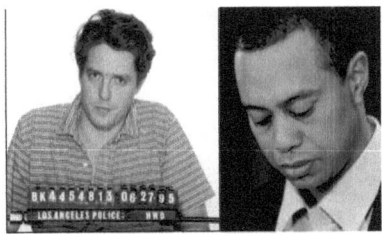

Hugh Grant, the famous British movie star can be an example; he is handsome; he has one of the world's most beautiful sexy women as his girl friend. He is an extremely talented as an actor. I have enjoyed his movies.

He had his scandal when some tabloid reported that he was caught with a sex worker in one of the lowest sections of town. In my mind, it was clear. He had had to do his chase, then conquer, feel the emptiness and then remorse and detach.

Pete had his opinions about this too. "Bryce, he is a handsome man who is desired by any woman you can think of. He is an international movie star. He has everything going for him." Then he asked a rhetorical question. "Why do you think that he did this?"

"I think that he was envious of other men doing it with a $25 prostitute in the dangerous streets of some sleazy part of town." I said. "I guess that he just wanted to have what he had not had. His reason must have been that maybe this will wipe off the emptiness that other acts of sex had not wiped out."

Pete was thinking the same way. He chimed in with "Just like Dean Martin thinking the next woman will satisfy him. The satisfaction that he had not found after all these chases that he had conducted!"

"What were you thinking?" David Letterman asked him in his show. "The answer was a simple 'I do not know' and they somewhat left it at that."

As a European, back in Europe he is judged by the European standards. These European standards are different from those of ours in US. Again, I am not judging, but they believe that private matters are to be private. Many countries by legalizing prostitution, have managed to reduce crimes related to illegal prostitution.

Pete had to jump in again. "Bryce, it is ironic that David Letterman himself had had affairs after affairs thinking the same thoughts!" Then as if sorry for some major lost opportunity, he said, "I wish I could see David Letterman's interview of Hugh Grant (or Grunt as the British accent sounds!) David Letterman must have been laughing his heart out. He, who was having affairs, was asking Hugh "What were you thinking?" I was thinking that I was not exempt from this mental disturbance either. For years I had that burning urge to have sex with those perfectly painted movie stars. For years I too had the Pavlovian style brainwash to think that the best thing in this world was to have sex with some movie star! I was convinced mentally, emotionally and sexually that that perfect sex with a perfectly looking woman was the thing to do. In fact that was the thing to do! That was the world's biggest and most important pleasure.

This is another example of overt American hypocrisy when it comes to matters sexual.

Rod Stewart of "Da Ya Think I am Sexy?" fame said that he has lost track of how many women he had gone to bed with. Just like others, he too pointed out that he missed his second wife who divorced him. This is interesting. Rod Stewart, who could go to bed with any woman that he wanted to, still was missing something. That something was the love of his second wife. Rod also admitted that he preferred blondes. When asked why, he explained that the sexiest women he knew were both blondes. These two women who had turned him on when he was young were Brigitte Bardot of France, and our own Marilyn Monroe. However, he added something that I had experienced too. He said, "The most attractive woman in the world will not turn him on with her beauty alone. She must do something sexy as well." For example, "she needs to wear her skirt too high or tease him with some sex talk. Otherwise, he will not be interested!"

Having said all of these, I was shocked to hear about Tiger Woods. I admire, envy, and respect him as the best of the best golf players. I still, put him on a pedestal when I think about him. He is bigger than life.

He has everything that one might imagine bring happiness. At least it looked like he had it all as he appeared in front of cameras and on golf clubs.

His parents seemed to have dedicated themselves to him. He had the best training and he had achieved what every professional golf player dreams of achieving. His wife is a world class, elegant, sexy, and attractive woman.

On one of my recent business trips to London, I decided to give myself a mini-vacation and visit Liverpool. Liverpool is the home of Beatles. Before they were famous, they played in Liverpool pubs.

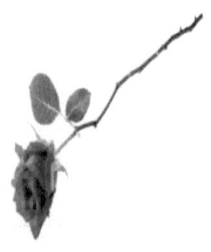

In fact a pub, or any pub, in the cold and wet city of Liverpool is a place to go after work and linger until later when the real night line goes into full swing. It seems like the town is painted by black as the dominant color. Nevertheless, as soon as you enter a pub and hear the music and cheers, you are instantly lifted up in spirits. For those few days, it seemed like I subsisted on "Pub Grub" which is the food that is served in these joints. In some the food would be fantastic. However, unfortunately in most the food would not be that good. Nevertheless people went there for the music and partying.

That first night, I was fascinated by so many attractive women in this particular pub that was only two blocks away from my tiny hotel. There also seemed to be fewer men than women. In some cases, the pub code of behavior dictated that once a man had started talking to woman, then that couple would be left alone. Other men would not try to make a pass at least while they were talking.

I met Jeanie this way. She worked in an office and lived with her mother who was quite till. They had a one bedroom flat and her father had passed away quite some time ago. Our conversations then started to revolve around intimate things. Considering that I had just met her, I was shocked at how much I had told her in the first thirty minutes.

She loved to cradle the wine glass and swirl it so ever gently from time to time. Her eyes had penetrated my soul and I felt quite helpless. I was mesmerized and fully under her control or spell. While this thought was very scary since she was a total stranger, I would calm myself down by telling myself that a woman who took care of his ill mother cannot be all that bad.

Inadvertently, after a few drinks and in a bar like this the subject of sex would come up. "How was the first time that you had sex?" is a starter. Then, "What was the strangest place that you had sex?"

Once this ritual is done, then "subject of what is next after the pub closing" comes up. As we were making progress in this part of the routine, her cell phone rang and she told me that she had to go. Her mother needed her. A fast goodbye followed by a sincere kiss. This convinced me that she was honest.

A few seconds later, I noticed that another business man was sitting next to me. His clean suite and nice tie were evidence that he was successful. "Hello, my name is Bryce" was what I needed to say just test the waters with this man. "Hello, I am Steve and you are from Chicago!" was his quick introduction to get the polite introduction over with so we can continue our search for the next one night stand. I noticed that his hair was shiny silver with some grey overtone. His gold reamed glasses looked like a professor. I realized that there has been too much time gone by without either of us saying anything. Acting supersized, I asked him "How did you know I am from Chicago?" He jokingly laughed it out by saying "A lucky guess". Then he became more serious and said that he was right behind me registering in the hotel. Our conversation got more and more interesting as time went by.

As if it was not enough for me to have told all my life history to the Jeanie, this man started an interesting conversation. He said, "I am Steve, and I am a sex addict!" This caught me by surprise. Why was he telling me this? My mind was going a thousand miles per hour. The idea of sexual addiction seemed to be strange to me.

I had a good understanding of drug and alcohol addiction, but sex addiction sort of still baffled me. The scene must have been completely comic to some observer. Two older men each over fifty and perhaps sixty are having what amounted in my mind to a juvenile discussion. I was feeling somewhat embarrassed.

Around 11:00 PM the bartender offered us a half priced drink that was the house special. It was a white wine from Napa Valley. Napa Valley, California wine which had came from half way around the world. I noticed he too was wearing a wedding ring. This made it easier for me to continue our discussions. Like me, he too had to be responsible. It is one thing when we were young and single and lived a wild life; it is a different thing when we are married.

Steve was originally from Toronto and had lived a few years in Chicago. Then, he moved to Cheyenne, Wyoming after he got married. He loved the nature and slower pace of life there compared to Chicago. I felt comfortable enough to ask him what sexual addiction really meant. "Simple, it is just like Alcohol. You have a drink and you feel good. Then that good feeling goes away sooner or later. Then you drink the next and the next. Eventually, you drink your work, relationships, and freedom away. Sadly, you keep thinking that you can stop any time you want. The horror is that you cannot, you have to keep drinking to be functional! I meant functional enough to cope with regular demands of everyday living! You just cannot stop; you want that next drink at any price!"

It was my time to share something with this trusted man. "I think about sex all the time. Does this make me a sex addict?" His response was "First men are wired to think about sex often. However, addiction is based on behavior not necessarily thoughts." Then he took a napkin and started to write something on it. He had drawn a map for a midnight sexual addicts' anonymous meeting that met every midnight. Before, he was going to write a phone number, I asked him if he was going there that night. "Of course!" he said. "Can I go with you?" His delighted answer was, "Of course!"

We shared a cab ride, and we were there a few minutes earlier. People started to introduce themselves as so and so and hen, "I am a sex addict" or "I am a sex and love addict". They shared the deepest feelings and talked about the most difficult things in their lives.

Totally out of the blue, I remembered my time in Red Light District. Was I a sex addict? At least, I was a sex addict during that period of time? Was a love addict? Why did I do what I did? I was deeply touched by this adventure side trip as part of my business trip. My mind drifted back to Chicago and my wife and children. I asked myself, "What would they think if they saw me here in this meeting?" Right next to me was a sex worker. She looked presentable and she had a pair of blue jeans and a nice blouse and a Scottish sweater. I knew she was a sex worker because she said that in her introduction. She was on step four of recovery which was taking an inventory. Her thick overcoat was carefully draping over the back of her seat not to touch the floor. She would make sure to check and adjust her overcoat. To my disappointment, she disappeared a few minutes before the end of the meeting.

Steve introduced me to a few others and it was time to go back to my hotel and call it a night. Before I could fall sleep, I looked at the thin phone book and noticed there were several escort pages. Next day I woke up with the phone book on the floor right next to my bed.

During the flight back, I read for the first time about the Tiger Woods' scandal. Why did he do this?

Maybe he was a sex addict and he did not know it. Maybe, he was not and all these things were made up. For that matter, maybe, I too, in the last quarters of my life have become a sex addict also. What was I thinking as a sixty year old man to act like a sex crazed juvenile? Most sixty year olds used to get ready for their retirement and playing with their grandchildren. There I was a law abiding and with Puritan upbringing who always fallowed the law to its strictest interpretation was acting out in Sheri's Ranch.

I had always admired Tiger for his golf genius. He was infinitely better than I. When he would do that perfect swing, it would be what I could only imagine even if I did not have lower back problems.

In addition for having golf in common, we have several other things in common too. We are both from families that had sacrificed part of their own lives to train us to become the best of the best. They wanted us to be successful, to be a good human being, to be an important person, to have ethics and honesty and all those qualities that a parent dreams in a good son or daughter.

In the most part, we were that good son or daughter that almost all other parents dreamed for their children to be. I for example had a perfect Math score at in SAT. Of course, compared to a global sports hero and champion, my accomplishments are nothing. To be that good kid, we did not hit other kids, we did not cheat in our exams, and we did not embarrass our parents. We made them proud. We made them happy each and every time another parent told their son or daughter look at Bryce, or Tiger, for being so, so good.

If the burden of being so, so good was killing us inside, we did not let it show.

I remember that each time I got anything less than the highest score, my dad would try to understand why and he would go to any extreme to help me get that perfect score the next time in that subject. I would spend a great deal of my time and life to never fail. At least never fail in Math and other things that were so important to my parents.

As a teenager, I did not do any of those things that teenagers did. If I went on a date, it had to be according to the French standards code of behavior. I was not supposed to have sex until after marriage. I was not supposed to even date a girl, unless I had clear intentions of marrying her. The date was to determine whether we made a couple capable of being happily married for ever after.

Although I was not told this, it seemed that I deep inside believed that sex had only one purpose and that was to procreate. After all I had read about those unintended pregnancies happening to most respected girls. I still remember an article about coat hanger abortions and sleazy South Side Chicago makeshift abortion so called clinics.

My folks did not have to tell me, I had known this instinctively.

No sir, I did not do those things! I was going to find the love of my life and marry her happily ever after. Unfortunately, one detail was left out. That detail is human nature. It is human nature to enjoy enjoyable things in the world. It is human to want to have fun in life. It is human nature to want to be like all others. We did see a lot of this in sexy advertisements on TV or bill boards selling chewing gum, milk, or cosmetics. The Hollywood and TV shows seemed to have had hopelessly brainwashed us that the biggest pleasure is to have perfect sex, in perfect setting, with the perfect woman and be the perfect man. Any shortcoming, any tiny human flaw was unacceptable! Then you could not get this. It was illegal!

So, what was a man supposed to do? Some got married to the wrong woman after that first fulfilling sex. Some decided to go abstinent. Some decided to ignore all and just have fun.

Just have fun!

I have a best friend who lives in Seattle. I called him last week. Jerry is married and has three kids. Kids are not quite right since they are all grown up and they have left the nest. However, golf is his love. In fact he got married in an exclusive golf club near Chicago before he left to live in Seattle.

"Hey Jerry, how are you doing." I asked him. "I am watching the Masters in Augusta. Tiger is back and I am hoping that he would win! Otherwise, I would be disappointed." This was Jerry's response. "But Jerry how can you expect this from a man who must have gone to hell and back this last five months?" was my reaction. In a dismissing way he said, "He always wins! He is the god of golf and I cannot accept anything less." After a sudden switch of subject, he asked, "Did you see that Nike advertising the other night?" He was referring to a black and white ad that tried to portray a remorseful Tiger by putting his father's voice asking him, "Tiger, what were you thinking?" Of course this was referring to him after having had affairs.

I knew the feeling that Tiger would have had right at that moment. I had felt the same when I came home with a score less than perfect. If I was Tiger, I might have revolted and said "What do you expect me to be thinking? I was a human being. I was a human being who is brainwashed to have pleasure by all the society and advertising media. I was not thinking right at that moment, I was trying to absorb, and be delighted in what I had seen as the most exciting thing in the world. The perfect sex with the perfect woman and being that perfect man! I was a human being, nothing more and nothing less! But do not expect me to be thinking when I was under the undue overwhelming delight that I was promised. "

Jerry had always been a voice of reason and sanity for me. In fact, he is the one who encouraged me to learn golf. He loved this game and he had several trophies. "Bryce, he was wrong to be unfaithful to his wife! He was wrong to do this even if he was not married. We must in control of our feelings and behavior at all times?"

For that moment, I was in agreement with him. However, the thought of having a few quarters to live had lifted a lot of my inhibitions and had made braver. It had made me braver to even do things that my Puritan ethics would have considered unethical. I had just a few months and then I was supposed to die. I had been told that sex can mean death to me because of heart condition. The blood pressure medications had rendered me "Nonfunctional in bed". Let us be clear, they had made me impotent. Impotence had forced me into being depressed. Combination of impotence and depression was telling me that I could not have that one and only best thing in the world. This had seemed to give me a decision to make between compliance and dying each day a bit more, and revolt.

I chose revolt! I was not dead yet. I decided to live and actually live it up!

Jerry's reaction to some of my thoughts was, "I can sort of understand. But Bryce, as a religious person, I cannot agree with you. I would not do these things if I were you."

As our discussion shifted to golf, as it usually did when I talked to Jerry, he quickly pointed out that Tiger must love his job, the job of playing golf as a living!" I seemed to have a severe reaction to this statement. "Jerry, we do not know this. Even Tiger does not know this! Did he actually have other careers? Did he really try something else? Did he dream about being a fighter jet pilot as a kid? Did he ever dream about being a fireman? Was it ever his ambition to be a cowboy? Did he do all those things that childhood is all about? Was he ever a kid, aside from golf?"

Jerry was going into this long winded explanation when I got distracted. I was totally distracted when I had silently discovered for myself that Tiger must have not had a childhood. Most of us go to many therapist sessions talking about our bad childhood. At least we had a childhood of some sort or the other. What if Tiger did not have any of that? What if he was reporting to his job of golf championship as early as when he three or four? More shocking to me was this question: Did Tiger have any choice?

From all I know, his parents loved him and he loved them. I caught myself. I was speculating that he must have had not been happy with his job. That had created some stress. Then the poor man must have had some difficulties in his marriage. We all have some difficulties in our relationships and marriage. He could not have been an exception. So, he was in a double bind. He did what any ordinary human being does. He sought an escape. He was like an alcoholic who decided to go to bar and have a last drink. This time he had promised and promised that this one will be indeed be the last drink. He needed some relief. He needed some relaxation.

"What do you mean by relaxation?"

It was Jerry, demanding to know what I was mumbling to myself and that he had finally locked into the word relaxation. As if talking down to a five year old, he objected, "Relaxation, my foot!" Tiger and his multimillion dollar sponsors do not play or get psyched up with golf. This is serious enterprise business! This is huge!"

After cooling down a bit he said "Sorry, I did not mean to offend you!" "Jerry, you did not offend me. You are right!" I had decided to call it a long day and retire to my bed that night. I had forgotten the main reason of my calling Jerry. I had called his, as I had called him hundreds of times before to ask him to be my sounding board. I was trying to figure out what he did if he had only a few quarters to live.

I guess that I never will find that one out. It seemed that at some point in my discussion with him, I had totally ignored all he was saying, or all that he was standing for. Then, I had effectively gone into this daydream. When I unconsciously realized that it was not nice to ignore my buddy, the word relaxation had exited my daydream stage and verbalized itself. This was in response to silence on the line when Jerry was hoping to hear something back after his lecture.

Would I have done what Tiger did? Suppose I was in his shoes. Would I have done the same things? The answer is maybe. Nevertheless, if the question is that would I have done things if I knew that I had only a few quarters to live, the answer would be a resounding yes!

"Wait a minute!" I was talking to myself. "What he did was illegal or at least unethical! You did not break any law, you just visited sex workers!" Self talk got more intense and forceful. "You were strictly legal according to Nevada law, when you were in Nevada on a connecting flight. You were ethical in that you did not charge your stay in Nevada to your company as a business expense and other cash register honest things that you have always done."

Tiger could have done the same to deal with his urge. He could have flown to Las Vegas and he could have gotten the same limo with your friend and confidant Warren. He could have asked for a line up. He could have picked one or even two or three of the sexiest women in the world and have had perfect sex with them. All safely and all in strict confidence! He could have afforded it. More importantly, nobody would have known about it.

I remember that on my second visit to the Ranch, Warren and I were talking about affairs. I had just read a complete book about it on my extremely long business trip from Singapore. Warren is one of the few that I can talk to about anything. His fatherly and friendly advice still remains with me even today. Right after he picked me up from McCarran Airport in Las Vegas, offered me my usual cold Iced Tea in long can. He even knew that I liked it chilled and lemon flavored. The drink was exactly that. As we started our forty or forty-five minute drive, I was eager to tell him about the book that I had just finished reading. It must have taken me five minutes of boasting and describing what I had read. Warren was listening and listening intensively. He was listening so intensively that he had asked me to repeat what I had said twice on different occasions. Then, I asked for his advice and insight.

"Bryce, I am not an expert in this subject. I have had great times in my marriage, and I have had bad times too. Just like anybody else. So, I will give you my advice and charge you exactly what it is worth, which is nothing!"

"I would not have an affair. If I had been tempted to must have had an affair, I would only consider having it with those who would have just the same to lose as I did. As a married man, I will never have an affair with a single woman. If discovered, it will cost me my marriage and it will cost her nothing! This is not a fair exchange." Then with a smile, he said "A word from our sponsors. Just come here and have the pleasure that you want. Get satisfied. Then go home to your wife and family without any fear of diseases or scandal." Just as if he had not said enough, he added, "As you know, advertising says what happens in Las Vegas stays in Las Vegas and we intend to keep it that way!"

This caused me to go into deep thought. I hated my job. It was stressful. My marriage was even more stressful. These visits were the only way I could relax. These parties were gifts that I had given to myself to stay alive in an already dead career and marriage while I was dying too!

I suppose, this would have not been enough if Tiger was also wanting to have the excitement of having an affair. Just sex was that one thing he was longing for. Unfortunately that only thing part of it had made it imperative that it must be an affair. Just sex with a sex worker would have not satisfied him enough. It had to be a dangerous affair. Actually, he longed to have that perfect affair just like that perfect game of golf that he was able to play. The perfection would have been a protection against being caught just like all these other stupid husbands. After all he was Tiger!"

This is where Hugh Grant seems to have something terribly similar in common with Tiger. Hugh was able to have sex with every woman that he desired. What was important was that he was not even married. So, nothing would have satisfied his longing, urging, need except for having that one and only thing.

This had to be nothing less than having sex in a car with a total stranger street walker. This meant taking the risk of contracting AIDS. This had to be taking the risk of being attacked by some gangs. In addition, this meant taking the risk of being attacked, or mugged at the gun point by the woman's pimp.

Perhaps, Hugh was convinced that he could get away with this because Hugh Grant was Hugh Grant!

Passion had blinded his ability to think rationally. Billion dollar Madison Avenue advertising had brainwashed him to go for the gusto, and to go for that perfect most important thing.

He did go for the gusto. Unfortunately, he got caught. And when he did, he lost and he lost big. Warren seemed to have been right about his theory about affairs.

That day, I had flown from Los Angeles to Las Vegas. We had to attend a face to face meeting in a conference room in a major hotel right next to LAX. Then, the local general manager had given me a ride to the airport just in about enough time to catch my flight to Las Vegas. The trip to LA was a total waste of time, as we all knew weeks before. The client had convinced himself not to buy our products and there was nothing to change their minds. Furthermore, several phone calls had proven to be going nowhere. So, my company had decided to send heavy guns this time. Heavy guns were me and my colleague Nathan. Nathan is a hell of conflict resolver. People love him. He is professional and he had had some really negative reactions to this trip. On our flight to LA, he had several times told me that he did not like to work with the "Corporate Whores" that were trying to get away with not paying for the contract that they had with us. Being experienced like I was, he too had determined that this was a last ditch effort by our company. Nevertheless, he was bitter. He did not want to work with this company.

We had carefully orchestrated our strategy. We know how much we could give in and how much we could not. We had the video conference call arranged for our executives and theirs to make sure we all understood the conclusion. When I heard the word whore from Nathan, I was perturbed. What did he really mean?

About half an hour before our flight landed in LA, Nathan repeated what he had told me earlier in the flight and I had not quite heard it. Nathan was emphatically telling me something very important this time. "Bryce, I will not prostitute my career, belief system, and faith. I will not lie to them. I will not try to tell them something that was not the truth, and the real truth." "Nathan, I will not prostitute myself and belief either. I will tell them the truth, but I will not tell them the part about our company sending us as a last ditch effort. I will not tell them that we knew darn well that we could not afford a long legal suit with them. I knew darn well that my superiors had already decided on this." Just to sooth his hurt feelings, I told him "Nathan, we are just workers. Just like any other workers. We have to put food on our table just like they have to do the same for their loved ones. It is just a job! It is just a daily work. It is not our lives. We do not intend to marry them; we just need to be true to our own truth as we see it during this three hour ordeal. This is like being a sex worker and not a whore. There is nothing more nothing less. We will be our own men after this just like we were before." Nathan had cooled down. He seemed to agree with me." Then just to make sure he was OK, I added that "I had a game of golf waiting for me right after this." He was curious. "Will you be playing golf in LA?" I had to carefully jump in and say, "No, no!" Hastily I told him that the golf game was waiting for me in London!

Wow, this was a close call. The golf game was not in London. It was at the Ranch. They do have a nice golf course right there. In addition there is also a nice yard that has a waterfall and a barbeque stand for special occasions or private parties. If Nathan ever figures out where my next destination is I will be in trouble.

It seemed like I had been transplanted to another time and planet thinking these thoughts. I heard Warren telling me "Your flight out of McCarran International is delayed by at least one hour. I checked before I left. I will check again while you are in there partying. It seems like this will give you some extra time to relax in our sports bar if you like. Otherwise, I can drive you to the airport earlier if you wish."

It is this professionalism that does impress me every single time.

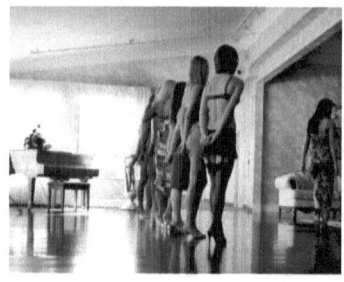

CHPATER 24: Sex Workers, Legal Brothels, and American Hypocrisy

My journey seemed to have had started with being somewhat innocent and perhaps naïve. If I was to have only quarters to live, then why not live it up?

I was not going to be like my dad with a lot of unfinished things while nailed to deathbed dying! As much as I loved my folks, I had realized much earlier that we were very much different.

I seemed to have a harmless violet wild side that they did not have. Unlike them, I would stand up to injustice. I would stand up regardless of the price I had to pay. In contrast, they seemed to be more reserved.

Being immigrants from elsewhere, their survival instinct would go into high gear the minute they had to object to some social injustice.

As a child, my parents taught me that "You do not Fight City Hall!" Now in my sixties and having had a serious performance problem in bed, I had relearned what I had learned in my twenties. I had learned that performance problem or not, I need to do what I had to do. I had to stand in picket lines in anti war rallies. I had to refuse to pay credit card balance that was more than ten times what I had borrowed from them. I was not just fighting for myself; I was fighting for all others who could not defend themselves. Being a first born, helps you effortlessly play this role!

I had obeyed the law to the teeth.

I had never visited a sex worker. Call it lack of courage; call it extremely high moral standards; call it whatever you want.

However, for more than thirty years, I had been conditioned just like a Pavlov Dog to have a burning desire for those graven images of perfect, air brushed, and made up women on bill boards, TV programs, and newspapers and magazines. I must admit that at times the urge was a lot more than I could handle!

My mind was totally programmed that there was only one thing, and one thing alone in this world and that was to win the sexiest woman in the world. When the man had finally managed to get woman in bed after heroics and perfection, then I would enviously dream of the same thing. I would wish to jump out of my seat in the movies and then somehow transport myself into the man that was going to have that perfect sex under perfect circumstances! That was Nirvana! If right there and then, the woman would change her wig, or just I notice the smallest of imperfection, then I was not interested at all anymore. This had happened again and again when I was at Sheri's Ranch.

It was time to call Pete and see how he was doing. I called him. He said that he was not feeling very good. He had to be hospitalized for three nights, and then he must have caught some virus there in the hospital that forced him to stay another two nights. He was elated that he had learned a new term. Bryce they call this "Hospital Acquired Condition." After a short laugh, he started to cough like crazy. "See, this is what I got while I was there. I caught flu!"

In spite his coughs, he was really happy that I had called. He told me "Bryce, I am really proud of you for getting this out of your system. If I had only a few quarters to live, I might do the same!" Then he disgustedly caught himself! "I would do the same things you are doing, if I was not chained to this damn wheelchair." I had to jump in the middle of his sentence.

"Pete, there is a ramp in front of the Sheri's Ramp just for this purpose!" He then with scolding, yet gentle voice said "You know what I mean! I should have done these things way before I got old!"

"Hey Pete, I too have learned new things!"

This whole sex thing is a viscous cycle. I see an attractive woman and I want to have sex with her. The urge gets explosively hot during the chase. Then the thrill of the chase does its trick, and I go to bed. Of course, this assumes that I had not suddenly lost interest because I had found some tiny defect.

Then moments after climax, I feel stupid, empty, and remorseful. Of course, I am satisfied and happy, but somehow some idiotic thing tries to spoil it.

I had felt this in the Red Light District as well as in Sheri's. Right after the act, I just wanted to get out of there and go home. The same woman who had ignited a sexual flame in my body and soul was now of not much interest any more.

In fact for those two or three hours after the act, I was not interested in any sex anymore!

"What, Bryce not being interested in sex anymore?" Pete commented. "Yes, that was the strong feeling!"

"So what if prostitution was legal in US?" "That way, I would have not tortured myself all these years with a burning urge for sex that could not legally be satisfied. But, illegally it was being satisfied all around me." I said to Pete. He seemed to want to make a point right there and then. "I agree with you. There might be less crime of passion. There might be less human trafficking. There might well be a lot less unhappy marriages. But, my religious upbringing says absolute no to legal prostitution!"

Somehow, the word "unhappy marriage" caught my attention. I had for the longest time tried to read books on what made a marriage happy. I had for many years asked couples that seemed loving about their secret to happy marriage. All of a sudden some spark of genius seemed to get my mind go in over drive. I started to think of marriage being a commitment for ever. Then, what if all of a sudden the wife says, no more sex! Or, visa versa?

The intense urge combined with illegality of visiting a prostitute then creates an impossible situation. As it happened many times before, it seemed like I had made Pete's point for himself. "Right, in those cases it really should be legal!" Then quickly he added, "It should be legal, clean, and healthy!" "But Pete, we are the only Western country that has made prostitution illegal." He was in agreement with me. He then started with some confirmations of his own. "I almost married a bartender under undue urge! Of course, I was also drunk at the time!"

I started to look outside my window and see that my wife's car was almost in front of the house. Her headlights had lightened up the falling snow. Otherwise, I would have tried to ignore the snow away. We had just had much too much of the white stuff that winter.

My wife's car is a station wagon Volvo. It has a navy blue exterior with one of the finest beige lather interior. She bought that car new without even telling me. The truth is that I would have told her that Volvos are reliable and safe cars. Nevertheless, she wanted to have done it all by herself and then surprise me. After years of marriage, I have learned to pick my fights carefully. I only fight for what is important. The fact that she had paid considerably more than that car was worth was not important in view of the pending divorce of all these years.

"Bryce, you mess with me just one little bit, and I will file right away. You know, I can take the kids, and the house!" She will mouth these things, and I would semi ignore them. Then, she will find something or other to fight. Then there will be a new day, and she might forget all of these. In a party with my manager, she was pretended to be very proud of and very happy with me. "I love this man!" she told my boss. Then, right after having said that she would loudly whisper in my ear "This will cost you, man this will cost you!"

The next day during breakfast, she would add that everything she said were lies and I should not let any of that nonsense to go to my fat head!

"See, all you men are like Tiger Woods!" "He has an excellent wife. Then he goes and has multiple affairs. I would have tried to kill him too! Men are just not good!"

With these thoughts still on my mind, I said goodbye to Pete and turned on the TV. I changed to sports channel. I used to watch sports channel most of the time before I had problems in bed. Now, with problems in bed, I tend to watch British Comedy, Direct channel from Paris with a weekly variety show that sometimes includes topless as if that was something "routine". I remembered the big deal that was made regarding "Wardrobe malfunction" when accidentally and only for a few seconds a breast was exposed on national TV here in the US.

I remember that my brother-in-law had gotten some very expensive final soccer tickets. Manchester United, one of the best football (European Soccer) teams was playing against the Spanish team. My brother-in-law and I had flown from London to Barcelona just for this game. Our return would leave Barcelona at Midnight.

We were so drunk that we did not even know who won and who lost. We should have been denied boarding. In fact, I am sure that had we been in an American airport, or trying to board an American flight, the crew would have taken one whiff and cancelled our tickets and even our birth certificates if they could due to intoxication!

I was sitting in 23F and anxiously waiting for the flight attendant to start the food and beverage service. A well manicured hand tapped me on the shoulder. It was a woman fan. She politely showed me her ticket saying that my seat is 3E and I am sitting in 3F! The eyesight of drunks is not so perfect. So, she probably was right. I offered that she could sit in my lap and that will correct the problem. She took a look and realized that the flight attendants were dealing with some other potentially drunks. So, with a nice voice and heavy British accent, she said "I, cunt!"

Unlike these days that cunt has an awful meaning, those days it was a sexy way of talking about a beautiful woman's "woman parts". She really meant, "I cannot!"

I was travelling at the speed of sound when I heard the word cunt. All of sudden, I remembered that when the Piano Teacher near Heathrow airport would tell me that she cunt have an appointment with me at 3:00, but that she can at 4:00. Then I will go over an hour agony thinking only about how much my man part needed and longed the company of her woman part.

In my latest trip to London, I had some spare time. These are called down times in our business and they usually happen when it is impossible to schedule meetings for some four to six hours. This breath of fresh air is cherished by business travelers and they take maximum advantage.

In one such rare occasion, I went to Harrods Department store. A white colored stripped Pierre Cardin shirt got my attention. Usually, this brand fits me well and the color scheme is a good match for my complexion. I found the nearest mirror and put the shirt near my face. I was sold! This shirt made me look awesome. Then I had to buy cuff links. I chose a real gold set that was really impressive. World class businessmen like me can easily tell if a cuff link is real gold or not. The real gold is a bit heavier and as such it makes the entire cuff look better.

A quick sandwich was enough to alleviate my hunger.

Earlier that day, I had noticed that I needed a haircut. Some of the new gray hair had diminished my Silver shinny hair's appeal. I saw a luxury men hair salon nearby and I went there. The owner, a Spaniard, assured me that he will be done in less than five minutes. I was Impressed to see he was done when he said he would be.

Then, with confidence, pride, and professionalism, he said "Would you like styling too?" I agreed to styling. Immediately I could tell that I was under the care of the best of the best. I appreciate and admire this. Therefore, it was a no brainer to agree to his suggestion that "Perhaps the gentleman would kindly allow me to take care of the gray by accentuating the natural silver color." He really did not have to ask, since I would have agreed to anything that he would say. After my hair was washed in preparation for styling, he asked, "May I offer a razor cut?" Razor cut is a lot more popular in Europe than it is here in the US. After cutting the hair to proper length, then a sharp razor is used to get rid of all those dead ends and make the hair a lot easier to maintain. I said yes before he could finish his sentence. I somehow knew and trusted that this man will do a masterpiece. I was right. My new styling haircut was so impressive that even he stepped back for a second and was deeply immersed in admiring his own masterpiece creation.

I looked and felt younger, sexier, and much more handsome than before I entered his barbershop.

I noticed that I had more time. I returned back to Harrods. I entered via the fragrance department which is world famous. A very sexy woman grabbed my full attention. "Sir, you might like our latest aftershave. It has a specially formulated scent that women cannot resist. Well, I heard this before. So, I did not pay any particular attention to this sales claim. That scent had permeated everywhere. Without even trying a sample, I purchased it and put it in the bag. As an afterthought, I had to admit that this aftershave had me made hot too.

Since I had bought a new shirt, it only made sense that I bought a matching tie. I noticed some fascinating ties from Scotland. My 12.5% Scottish inheritance lead me to a Pringle 100% silk tie that seemed was tailored just for me and that Pierre Cardin shirt.

A short stop in the china department to buy a teacup set for my daughter completed my pampering shopping spree. I had called her and made sure that this was exactly what she needed to complete her collection.

Where was I? I was at that flight after the Manchester United game. My brother-in-law, after having had done me the great favor of telling me about his affair with some beautiful lady had shook me up. I asked, "Affair? How could you have an affair? But you are very religious!" Then as if none of that was important, I insisted on him answering the next question. "Does your wife know?" I interrogated him.

His honest response was "I do not know!" I resuming where I had left my interrogation asked him. "How long ago was it?" His reply was baffling. Then, it seemed like he had just sobered up for a few seconds to share one thing. He added, "We have a three year old son together!" I could not believe any of this. Next day back in a London hotel, we met for breakfast. Before I could say anything, he said "Sorry for having made you worry last night. I was drunk. What did I really tell you? Please tell me!"

After a moment of rest, I thought "Good, there is no son, no affair, and no nothing. He was just plain drunk!" My peace and quiet got shattered when he started again and said, "Yes, I do have an illegitimate son. He does not even know what illegitimate means, but he is." Then a series of confessions followed. "I wish that I was dead! I wish I had never gotten involved with this hot woman."

My one track mind went back to the argument that if we made prostitution legal, then there would be less of illegitimate kids as well. He had one more thing to say. "If you say a word of this to your wife, my dear sister, or my wife, we both would be dead before we know it!"

Trying to keep my composure, I told him that he needs to get sex therapy. His objection hit the roof. "What sex therapy?" "That is another American hypocrisy!" A few seconds went by and then he said "Sex is what you do and feel, not what you talk about!"

"I spent many years sitting on a therapist chair and did not really get much. Sure, the hidden assumption is that everybody has some childhood trauma that triggers depression, or some other dysfunctional behavior. Then, it is also assumes that the therapist discovers what had happened, and helps the person with some simple steps to resolve the internal turmoil and trauma. It is as simple as that. Step one, two, three and bingo problem solved. Jackpot! Just like the movies and TV. It seems as easy as taking candy from the baby. Whoosh, and the problem is solved and everyone is happy. Magic wand is waved and the problems are gone forever. The classical case of happily ever after."

After a hurried gulp of water, he continued his tirade. "I cannot understand marriage counselors either. In most cases, they see their job as expediting a divorce. In their minds, there is a simple axiom. A bad marriage has to be ended. The sooner this happens, the better. In many cases, a divorce not only does not help, it even hurts more. Kids are the number one victim of a broken home. For God's sake, either call this divorce counseling. Let us be honest about this. I saw a so called marriage counselor for more than a year. Each time I went there, I got angrier. Each time I went there, there was the hidden or implied message that divorce is the solution. He fueled my fire of hatred and outrage."

After a long and deep seated pause, he was ready to put something else on the table. He has had it with this life. If divorce is the solution, then as the theme song in M*A*S*H movie is right too. One of the lyrics of that song says, "Suicide is painless!"

I had started to listen to him doing my best to be nonjudgmental. In fact I was quite ambivalent at the beginning. However, much to my disappointment of myself, I started to agree or at least see some of his points of view. I had been smart enough to do my "hands on" sex therapy in Red Light District and Sheri's Ranch. A generous gift from my best friend had bank rolled my world wind escapade of having sex with world class and most sexy women in the world. I had quenched my thirst in perfectly legal and so called victimless crime of prostitution. Shockingly, I could see that without having had outsmarted the system, and having had the means to do it, I too would have ruined my life and that of others. A night of careless sexual pleasure can result in complicated affairs, pregnancies, and even life threatening AIDS and other things. The porn that is pervasive everywhere, does not show this side of things. Unfortunately, kids who are results of such indulgences will end up living life with a single parent. These kids most likely end up being scarred for life.

Even though I had managed to successfully and totally tune out what was being said to me with great urge and intensity, I realized at this point that I had to start listening again.

I could see the rage in his eyes saying these words. At the same time, I could see the deep sorrow and sadness that must have taunted him for years. While his rage was brewing inside he tried to make things more clear to me by saying "Bryce, you might have forgotten the flaming passion that will not leave you alone. Maybe you do not remember the time when you were twenty or thirty and had these urges. I had them since I was fourteen. I am no psychologist, but I have read that everything we think and do goes back to our sexual desires. Was it not Freud who said this?"

Then a barrage of words came out of his mouth that even surprised him after he had said them. He said "I drink because I feel lonely, unloved, untouched, and unwanted. I drink instead of sex and love. Liquor tends to squelch my urge for sex and love; at least it defuses it and reduces my pain for a while. I know the damn thing is destroying my liver and my life, but I do it anyway."

Then, as if trying to be friends again, he reminded me that his affair would have never happened had he gotten enough sex and intimacy at home with his wife. In fact, he was still fighting with his wife. He was fighting he first wife who had divorced him many years ago. That unexpected divorce had pushed him on the verge of total financial and emotional collapse.

Having thought these, I quickly realized that his first wife divorced him because he was a practicing alcoholic. Even when he was not drunk, his temper would flair up from time to time and create dangerous situations for him and others. It did not take a lot for him to lose his temper and go into a full fledge rage.

I had learned years earlier that the best way not to get hurt is to leave the danger zone while it was possible and before getting entangled! Pretending that I had a meeting that I had to get to, I said goodbye and rushed to the "Underground" which is the British word for our subway.

Once back in the serenity of my hotel room, I took a quick shower and ordered a modest dinner that turned out to be quite expensive. Thanks God for business accounts reimbursing these expenses. Even after the shower, I was feeling dirty. I could not put my finger on it, but I just felt totally out of place. I did not really know what I was doing with my life. I was not happy with my career, my marriage, my church, my friends, my health, and everything and nothing.

At the age fifty-eight, I was feeling all the aches and pains that this age has to bestow upon us. However, I was feeling sex, love, affection, and intimacy deprived and horny just like a fourteen year old. On top of that I was also feeling extreme anger towards my conservative upbringing. Wow, this was something; I was in three ages at the same time and felt like a rebellion teenager that was conflicted and confused.

Confusion was about sex at the beginning, then that painful emptiness expanded to overpower my entire life. Out of total harassment, disgust, and desperation I dialed my wife's phone. I had to talk to somebody. As far as I was concerned even a telephone operator would have been just sufficient. I needed somebody, I could use anybody. My wife's cell phone forwarded my call to her voice mail without even ringing.

I thought, "That is better. She will not know my anguish and pain. Why bother her? She has enough on her plate. I had missed all parent teacher meetings except two the last two years. She is a single mom for all practical purposes. I am an excellent provider, but an absent excellent provider." My executive salary had provided for new cars and private schools. Unfortunately, my distance and being on business trips more than fifty percent of time had taken its toll."

I fell asleep without setting my alarm clock or asking the front desk for a wakeup call. I was tired, homesick, horny and desponded.

I woke up at 5:00 AM GMT. My eyes were red and burning as a result of sleep deprivation, and my soul in pain. BBC World News was about half done when they did review of top stories. There had been another bombing in Northern Ireland the night before. Then, there was a report regarding the "American States of Illinois and Michigan". These two states had suffered record snow fall and massive blackouts as a result of storms and ice.

This seemed to add urgency to my return trip to Chicago. Too much had happened and I wanted to be home. I rushed packing and taking my laptop computer and getting downstairs to check out and get the cab to Heathrow airport. That day the infamous London fog seemed to feel sorry for me and thus hide itself. I was at the airport a full three hours ahead of the departure time. This is stupid. I had never been in the airport that early.

United Airlines representatives were not handling my direct flight to Chicago yet. It was just too early. However, a senior representative offered an alternative. I could take an earlier flight with a stopover in New York that would get me back in Chicago about an hour earlier. I decided against that and went directly to the lavish airport hospitality room reserved for business travelers like myself.

Our takeoff from Heathrow was smooth and uneventful. In less than thirty minutes we were flying high enough over Atlantic that I could no longer see the wave caps. Soon we were flying over the clouds and I fell asleep.

As my Being 747 was vibrating and jarring from left to right, I carefully looked at my watch that was set to local Chicago time. I was being pushed slightly to the left and then to the right all the time. This is not good news. I did not deserve this. After all, I had made peace with the Chicago O'Hare gods of winds many, many, years ago and had made them offerings of peace so as not to be subjected to this. They seemed to have reneged on their promises. It was as if they too were just as angry as I was and they were taking their anger and dread on poor me this time.

Captain with a confident voice came on the intercom system telling us that there is severe weather reported all around Chicago Land. There is heavy snow activity and visibility is poor. However, he assured us that the 747 was well equipped and that it should be able to land. Just be patient please! Then he asked the flight attendants to go back to their seats. This is another bad signal that a frequent traveler can easily understand.

About five minutes after this, we heard, "This is your captain and we were given a conditional permission to land. However, if we cannot land in one try, we will be diverted to another airport. As I mentioned there is severe weather activity at O'Hare!"

There seemed to be a complete whiteout. I could not see anything from my window.

In less than a minute, the captain was speaking on the intercom again saying that the flight right before us, a DC10, had had to abort landing due to unexpected wind shear.

Among most awful things that scare a passenger, wind shear must be on the top of the list.

The Captain hurriedly announced, "We are getting ready to land!"

The winds were tossing our plane sideways and sometimes pushing it a few feet up, and then let it go down a bit. I quickly became super religious and frantically cited my prayers. I loved these prayers that I had learned in my church when I was a child.

I could faintly see a tiny runway light. Right at that moment the fully leaded 747 was whooshed up a foot or so, and tossed to the left. The captain revved the engines and corrected this misalignment just in time. Then, like a hammer being slammed down, the right set of wheels and the front wheel finally rolling on the runway. In a fraction of second the remaining set of tires were dropped on the runway concrete. There seemed to be a premature applause by the passengers that was instantly muted as the captain had to activate the reverse thrust on engines full force. A nauseating worrying feeling overcame me.

Full application of brakes did gradually and grudgingly bring the gigantic plane to slow ambivalent stop.

One look out the window, and I had met my old worst enemy the whiteout condition! I could not see anything. Pretending that this was not so important, I rushed to the parking lot, got the shuttle bus and went to the long term parking. Dug up my car and started to drive. I was going to get back to my home and sleep in my own bed even if that killed me.

I really did not care! I wanted home.

Complete death of any communication, intimacy, or even care between my wife and I was even thicker than this eerie whiteout. She did not even care which flight and when I got home, or even if I got home at all. I suppose years of marriage and her going through the menopause has had its effect. However, as a gentleman that I was, I always posted a copy of my itinerary on the refrigerate door. My daughter usually reviewed that and she kept informed. She used to call me and ask for some sort of souvenirs depending on where I had gone to. Then upon arrival, my wife would protest that "I see you brought dust collector items again! Why do you do this?"

My thoughts went back to Las Vegas and its near perfect balmy sixty three degree temperature and was partially sunny. I pretended Gabriella, Kat, and Angelina were all present. Kat was carefully sipping coffee, Angelina was drinking her red wine, and Gabriella was enjoying her Cognac. I was having a telepathic conversation about the psychology of depression with Gabriella as she was caringly listening and validating my feelings.

In the absence of physical intimacy and sex, this had to do on a Chicago highway during one of the worst storms.

All of a sudden I noticed that there was a blinking detour light. I had just started to swear as loud as I could when the car in front of me came to a totally unexpected stop. In spite my years of experience in Chicago driving, I could not help banging into him. It was what is called a kiss. Most likely it had not caused any damage. I was positive that the driver in front of me must have felt this rear end kiss. To my outmost admiration, he did not even bother to stop and check. He just continued. His car was a lot newer than mine. I had rust in front of my car as a result of frantic over salting of highways in the winter. The excessive salt had eaten into body of my car. I turned on the inside light so the driver, whoever he was could see me. I then gave him a military salute to thank him for not making a big issue about the kiss. He returned the favor and did the same telling me graciously that he had accepted my thanks.

After a few minutes of solace, my battery light started to faintly come on!

This was unexpected. For years I had trusted and gotten excellent results from Sears' Diehard battery notorious for being an excellent match for horrendous Chicago winters. I told myself, "The hell with it. Since the alarm light was not fully on yet anyway, so I wished it go away. Miraculously the light turned off all by itself." Right at that moment I felt like a conqueror.

Soon I was driving on the detour. This time, the battery alarm came on in full force and persistently challenged me not to ignore it. I saw a liquor shop very close by. To my utter dismay and frustration it was closed. A dangling worn out "CLOSED" sign was unmistakenly visible.

I started to panic. After driving for another five minutes, I noticed a Dunkin Donuts shop with several cars in the parking lot. As if pushing a car that was just about ready to die any minute, I managed to barely park it as near the entrance as I could.

There was a warm and friendly atmosphere inside. Fresh brewed coffee was ready to be served and many fresh donuts were beautifully put in plain view in the show cases. I heard a customer request, "Sophie, could I get another refill?" and then "Coming right up!" was Sophie's response.

I could not believe my eyes. Sophie was superbly attractive. She was a tall natural blond with piercing blue eyes that most beautifully accentuated her white complexion. Her hair style with that breathtaking blonde hair was as if it was specially styled for her by the most exquisite Paris hairdresser. Her makeup was fresh and extremely well color coordinated. It seemed like she had just came out of a shower.

Her eyes were the most poetically gorgeous eyes I had ever seen. I sat on the counter fantasizing as if I could make love to her. She noticed that I was totally absorbed in her beauty. She gently poured some coffee for me and noticed my appointment book that was sitting right next to my hand. She asked "Are you on business travel?" That started a one hour conversation. She was smart and she read several newspapers each day. As the closing time neared I made sure that I had her phone number and planned to call her out. Closing time hit before I knew it. I was longing for her. She was attractive and intimate even with a total stranger like me.

As I left the Dunking Donuts shop I was hot for her and her intimacy. I wanted to cream her donut. I wanted to kiss her beautiful romantic lips that had come very close to mine when she pour coffee for me. I was going crazy. I wanted her so bad that I could not take it anymore.

The car made a semi-dead mocking bird noise as I tried to start it again.

A ton of bricks hit my soul. My mental voices and committees came alive yelling "Bryce, your Diehard battery dyeing on you is the least of your problems. You live in a La La Land. You were flirting and making mental sex with Sophie while you should have had to worry about your car. How stupid can you get?"

"Man you are almost sixty. Haven't you had enough sex?
Grow up man!"

It was true that there were more than my car batteries that
were dead. I was trying to have fun and forget not knowing
who I was and why I was even here. Like other man I too was
thinking about sex every five minutes. However, there is time
and a place for everything. Sophie is most likely married and
even happily married. She has her life and you have yours.

I told myself "Bryce, you will be pushing daisies soon. Get off
this childish romantic thoughts and passionate burning
desires. It was wrong for you to go to Las Vegas in the first
place. Maybe you should have never met or even felt or
touched any of those world class sexy and perfectly beautiful
women. Apparently doing this has hurt your life!"

I tried to turn the engine on again to no use.

I heard a tapping on the side window of my car. I had just
rolled the window just slightly down when I could not help
but get a whiff of a perfume that I was familiar with. It was
Sophie! Her perfume had turned me on when I was sitting on
the counter.

"Bryce, before I go, I noticed your car is not starting do you
want me to jump start it?" I was burning with desire. "Sophie,
do not just stand there. Come on in so we can figure out what
to do." Her blushing answer was "OK but just for a few
minutes, and then I really have to go!"

No sooner she had sat in my passenger seat that I gave her a
kiss on her cheek. She did not seem to be bothered by that. She
pretended that that had not happened. To change the subject,
and somewhat not knowing what will happen next, she said
"Look we need to get you going." I then politely asked her if I
could hold her hand. "OK if that makes you happy."

Without any hurry, I gently put my hand over hers which was resting on her beautiful thigh. Her skirt was made from some sort of satiny like material that flamed all my desires for her with outmost intensity. Then I heard her whisper "Hell, it is futile to resist." Then she gave me a kiss. It was a real kiss. My hand was caressing her beautiful hair when we had our first amorous French kiss. Several others followed in quick succession. By then my right hand had left her hand and I was touching her. I found her donut to be pulsating and delightfully warm."

Then somehow, my mental committee had the upper hand. "Bryce what if your wife finds out?" "Bryce you do not know who she is! Bryce this is unprotected sex. Worse yet, this is anonymous sex. You just met a total stranger. It is dangerous man! Stop it, stop it right now! I order you to stop!" Sophie's resonating and moaning voice at that moment was convincing enough to encourage me that I had her permission. Just to make sure I was no longer scared, she said that she had not had sex for over three months and that she was hot to trout. Then she gave the assurance that "You will be satisfied! I want you! I want you inside me! Go for it!"

I was "in there" as Warren would say, for more than an hour. We were exhausted and really deep down satisfied. I had not only creamed her donut well, but I had also creamed her panties! I could feel it."

As we were resting with her head on my shoulder, she said, "Bryce, this was the best I ever had!" Then she said that it will never be the same ever again. She was engaged to be married soon to a man that she loved and adored. Then as if not trying to hurt my feelings she added, "This was my bachelor party, a party that I will never forget. Then it was her turn to kiss me on the chick."

I was totally satisfied and fulfilled and invigorated.
Nevertheless there was a question that I was dying to ask
Sophie. "Sophie, what made us explode simultaneously in this
sexual panacea?" Then looking her into eyes, I pleaded as only
one lover can to another, "What did you see in me? What
turned you on? Why me? How? Please, please tell me the
truth!"

This had baffled her for a second. Then with a slow start and
guardedly she said "I had not had sex for more than three
months. I felt deprived and not alive. None of the donuts shop
customers turn me on. They are local and nothing like you.
You are a class act and world class businessman." She then
started to talk a bit faster. "By training I am a fashion designer.
So, you caught my attention with your real gold handcuffs and
the Pierre Cardin's latest shirt design. But, the thing that swept
me off my feet was your sexy aftershave. I just could not resist
it. I was aroused right after you sat at the counter and I could
inhale the scent. It turned me on right away. It was a strong
turn on." Then came one last installment, "Bryce, a sensitive
and caring man can be extremely sexy in the eyes of a
woman."

After a moment of silence and a passionate kiss, she confessed
to yet another thing. "Somehow the word Heathrow makes me
horny. I could not take it anymore when you said see you at
Heathrow next Monday at 8:30 AM GMT!"

My cell phone was ringing. It was my wife. She was asking
where I was. She did not know if I had made it to Chicago
from London. Sophie reached for my hand and so ever gently
touched it. I was satisfied and fulfilled. I was talking to my
best lover ever and my rough and difficult wife at the same
time.

By now Sophie patiently waited for the call to end. Then she
French kissed me again and said that she really had to go. This
time she really had to go.

It was faintly daylight.

She jump started my car. Then she gave me another hug and one last French kiss, ran to her car and speeded out of the parking lot.

My phone rang again. It was a record being called twice in a row. This time it was my son. Dad, pleas drive carefully. "We want you home alive" was what he was lovingly telling me.

I was alive OK. I was alive and burning with desire and passion. I had just made love to the most beautiful woman and hottest woman on earth.

I took a few wipes and started to clean myself after this heavy love making. I was totally wet. I had barely managed to clean myself that the car died again. I knew there was no hope of restarting it again.

I was stranded there for a good half hour when a Highway Patrol car stopped by. "Sir, what seems to be the problem?" He tried to jump start and it did not work.

We abandoned my car there and he gave me a lift to nearest motel.

This time, I was missing Sophie, and strangely enough, I was also painfully missing my wife. I had to re-examine my own sanity. "I asked myself if I was talking about my wife, my frigid, unfeeling wife." The answer came quickly. I must have gone crazy". Maybe this love making with Sophie was so passionate that it had burned the fuse on my brain. I was convinced; it must have done just that very same thing.

Even though I was totally and completely fulfilled, I caught myself searching for Sophie's phone number. After all I was a man and I was convinced that men never ever have enough sex! I wanted to get some more right there and then in that motel and with both Sophie and my wife. "Here you go again. You just mentioned your wife. She never was intimate with you. She never satisfied you. So, what is this nonsense all about?"

I had managed to get a few hours of sleep just to make a head start on that jetlag that was complicated by heavy partying that I started to remember something that I had seen in Sheri's Ranch website and their literature. Many of the women had indicated that they would also party with couples. In fact warren had told me that many married couples come here. I had not taken that seriously.

Maybe, I go back to Sheri's Ranch with my wife. Maybe they can cure her from this frigidity. Maybe they can rekindle a sexual passion fire that never ever was there. I kept asking, maybe, maybe, maybe.

I remember a song in the sixties and seventies that said something like "Call me an angel in the morning, an angel of the morning, angel".

Sophie had indeed been my angel of not just the morning, but life all together. She had resuscitated me back to being alive and feeling by her French kisses. As I was looking around, I found her lipstick smudge on the corner of my glasses. This ignited my passion. Like a heroin junkie, I turned the room inside out trying to find her phone number. The harder I tried the less I succeeded. I was horny and furious. I was turned on, anticipating and longing. I could not resist. I had to make love to Sophie one more time. I needed to make love to her just one more time. I just could not get used to not having her. I wanted to have her, even if it was for just one last time. This time, I would have wanted to have sex and make love to her until the daybreak.

I was feeling so lonely that I was trembling. My blood once boiling with passion when I was with her had ran ice cold. It was now or never, I had to find her for one more passionate sex. Maybe, if I made perfect passionate love to her, that alone would convince her to marry me instead of the guy she was going to marry.

These were tremendously powerful thoughts and feelings that were uncontrollably gushing out of my entire being. As each of these thoughts and feeling spewed out, I would have a rainbow of sensations. Fantasizing sensations that included, but were not limited to, pain, sorrow, remorse, egotism, erotic pleasures, sin, shame and blame, romance, nostalgia, imagination, and even envy.

The scent and sense of nostalgia lingered in my overheated imagination. It was clear that nostalgia came from Roya. I think that forever, I will wonder if marrying Roya would have brought us eternal marriage bless.

Depressingly, in the pit of my stomach, I had overwhelming pain. I understood this pain as one can understand a friend of many years. I understood that pains that I can see are not always as burningly painful than those that I cannot see.

The ecstasy of this intense sexual pleasure with Sophie had slammed open the doors to my closet of buried pains of the past. Now, in the last quarters of my life, sex with an infinitely sensual and irresistible woman had triggered a tsunami of painful feelings that had to be felt and dealt with. I had no choice. It was a life and death thing right before my death.

Shakiness was coming up. I was irritable, impatient, and aggravatingly agitated, restless, and depressed. Just like a crack cocaine addict, devastated, and homeless in some shooting gallery in some abandoned house I needed to get my next fix of Sophie.

The shooting gallery vision of myself inundated me with an avalanche of shame and blame that was fatally explosive and combustible as a mixture of isolation, self-centeredness, and addiction can concoct. Yet, I was doing the best I could to internally pull myself together.

"Bryce, you are one hell of an ungrateful bastard!" "You just had felt instant gratification with one of the most beautiful and sexy woman in the world. Be grateful! Many men would give their lives for such pleasure." My mental committee was trying to console and sooth my hurt feelings of pain.

Melancholy must have set in a few fractions of a second right after these calming thoughts had entered my mind. A screaming and horrifying thought crashed into my wounded and tired mind "Bryce, your crack cocaine is Sophie! You have to have one last fix. You must get this last fix or you will die. Unlike Methadone treatment available to crack cocaine addicts, your urge and longing for Sophie has no treatment. You must just get her. Get her one more time, and I promise that you will be free from you addictive dependency on her." I went back to bed before having made it to the bathroom to take a shower. It was a Saturday, and I did not care to sleep late. In fact for that matter, no one else cared either.

It was around 11:30 AM that sun came out for a brief minute from underneath ominous, thick dirty unfeeling cold black clouds.

I gave one more college try to finding Sophie's phone number. Unfortunately, I failed again. I thought about going to the donut shop, but she had told me that she would be gone for three days visiting parents in Schaumberg Illinois. Too bad I did not know her last name. Otherwise, I would have searched the entire Schaumberg Illinois to find her for just one more kiss.

My internal mental committee was shouting "Man, get real. Man, grow up! Man, are you crazy? You are old enough to be a grandfather, why are you doing these crazy things that a fourteen year old be tempted to do? Even a fourteen year old has more self control not to be so stupid!" In some poetic yet sadistic way I had to have what I wanted to have. I could not get over this fix. It was even stronger than alcohol, drugs, and any other substance. I had had intimacy, sex, and love in a short period way above and beyond my wettest dreams.

Like a teenager totally obsessed with sex, I drove to Schaumberg. In the first coffee shop, I found a phone directory of Schaumberg. Thanks God that compared to Chicago, this directory looked thin. I started from the first page looking for all listings of people with the first name Sophie, Sophia, or just S. I systematically and methodically underlined all.

Just like an alcoholic who had missed drinking, my hands were beginning to shake. I was dying for the intimacy, sex, and thrill of search. Maybe I propose to marry her right before I explode in a climax as I did the last time. "To do that, I had to find her before the wedding! Therefore time was of a big essence. It was now or never, and I had to have what I was absolutely supposed not to have!"

I then went to the nearest bank and asked if I could have change in coins for $100 to use a public phone . I carefully stacked up the change needed for calls and started to call. Hours went by. I was not deterred. I had to have what I had to have. Maybe, this will be one last time. But, I had to do this if my life depended on it.

Night fall arrives early in the winter time in Midwest. So, it was dark already around 5:30 PM. I realized that I had not checked out of the motel yet.

I returned to the motel and got some fast food along the way. By the time, I had gotten to the last names starting with letter "E" I fell asleep with my suit and tie still on. Needless to say, that I had a passionate dream about Sophie. It was all about Sophie. I could not wait to see her again. Maybe give her just one hug. Maybe, just so I get a chance to say goodbye. Not really, I wanted to make marathon love and have sex with her for just this one last time. Or, maybe, by marrying her, then we could have sex every night and it will be as passionate forever and ever.

The combined sobering effect of knowing that I might never find her and slight sanity instantly converted intense passion and hot desire into torturing remorse. I had been on this gut ranching sexual emotional roller coaster ride many times before. What masqueraded as a temporary sanity, splashed wave after wave of shame and blame tsunami! "Do you think Sophie will ever fall in love with you? She is love with somebody else. For God's sake she is marrying someone else! Bryce, come to your senses! Wake up and smell the roses!" This self talk designed to humiliate and defeat my self confidence plaid in my mind over and over again.

In passing, I remembered that Sophie had told me that her parents were very affectionate towards each other. She had told me that they would take pride in being sensual, intimate, and great partners to each other. Suddenly, these thoughts catapulted my mind into a nirvana-like thought. I thought that if I was married to Sophie, and only then, I would know what an intimate and sexually satisfying life could mean. Better than that. I would feel it once or twice each night long. Then, I would be happy and relaxed. Perhaps that relaxed attitude would have made me a better parent.

Sophie had intimated with me that she is the only daughter and she had three brothers. So, as such she had learned how to deal and even appreciate boys and men. Being the middle child, she had been given love by siblings older and younger than her. She was superb in relating to the opposite sex in an understanding, respectful, and caring way. My deductive powers then quickly arrived at a sour regrettable conclusion. The contrast and the devastating conclusion was that Dian was the total opposite. She had several sisters and one spoiled brother. Dian had told me several times that "All men are dogs and the best that should happen to them is to cut their man thing off. By cutting their man thing off, then they will leave us women to live in peace!"

This stinking thinking goes even further. Dian's best friends are Linda and Edna. Linda, whose parents divorced when she was only five, feels the same appalling feelings towards men. She is attractive and she dresses provokingly sexy. She has flirted with me several times. The painfully sad thing about her is that she is extremely uncomfortable with sex and intimacy. Her husband who lived under the same roof with her for more than fifteen years would be turned on by her and then repulsed and dejected right away. Finally, she filed for divorce. Edna, on the other hand is from a strict and religious family. Her mother and father were separated ever since she was twelve. Her father lived in an apartment about half a block away. Although for many years Edna and other kids did not know it, their dad had become addicted to gambling. So, each trip to casinos all around the country would result in one night stands with bar girls, card dealers, and bar tenders that he could wine and dine and have sex with. His mercurial temper usually would flare up and convince the girls to hit the road at least for their own physical safety. Edna honestly thinks that sex is dirty and it is just for a man's gratification. Edna's husband once had told me that all Edna knows about sex is "passive mission position!" He added with a great deal of anger that she spreads her legs, and then says something to the effect, "Please get it over quick!" She has complete disdain for the sexual act and she does not feel anything. Then her husband added with some brutally clear hatred that "Right after sex, I have to run downstairs to take a shower as if I had just been covered with dirt and dust."

The truth is that I do not like Edna's husband. He has on occasions hit his kids. He believes that unless kids are disciplined regularly, they turn into monsters and brats just like him. His pretzel reasoning is that since his parents were the permissive kinds, he never learned the value of discipline or respect for parents for that matter. So, as his reasoning goes, he blames everything that is wrong to this fact. I do not agree with this.

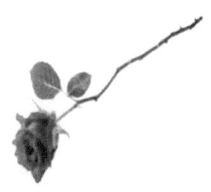

I was being pulled into two opposite directions. I felt like calling 911and reporting him as a child abuser, and, I felt sorry for this beast who was stupid enough to think this way. However the fact remained that these misfits always attracted Dain like a magnet.

My mind had drifted to many thoughts. It was time for me to go back to earth. I was becoming unstable. I could not think straight. I felt like I was having a fever.

There was a knock on the door next morning. Unshaved and in bad need of a shower, I saw that it was my son and daughter and I slowly opened the door. My son was horrified. "Dad, you do not look too good. Are you OK? Mom had called many motels to find this one and she had insisted that we had to come here to make sure you are OK."

This was a first. My wife never cared if I was dead or alive. She was too preoccupied with herself to care for me. She did however, love her kids dearly. She was a loving and caring mom.

"So, did she really send you?" I asked with a bit of disbelief. In unison they both said no. I knew my kids. I knew they were telling me the truth. "But dad, there is something that we need to tell you. Dad, there is something that we had decided not to tell you when you were in London on a business trip. We did not want to create panic." I did panic right at that point. "What, please, please tell me?"

There was a long thick suffocating silence in the room.

"Dad, mom had a car accident. She was in a five car accident hours after your flight had departed to London. Her Mercedes SUV was declared totaled. "My heartbeat hit the roof. "What are you telling me? How bad was she hurt?" Then my son broke out in a boasting description of the events. I could not hear much of that. Then while I was listening more intently to him, I heard him say "She spent two nights in the Intensive Care Unit. However, she was released two days ago!"

I had a combination of hurt, genuine love, anger, and disbelieve gushing into my awareness. "Let us rush home. I have to see her now!"

On the way home, riding in my son's car, my entire less than happy and fulfilling marriage played on and on in my mind. It was a love story combined with a horror show. It was enticing, informing, and yet sad.

One thing that I had learned from years of therapy was that, "Mr. Condon, this is the wife that you had decided to marry! No more no less!" Thinking with myself, I also added that this is the woman who gave me my kids. This was a strong "Here and Now episode of life's hard and cold calculating reality! She was who she was. I was who I was. The marriage was what it was at that moment. The world was what it was. I had to take these heavy dosages of what everything was, what they were right then and right there. There was no alternative choice. I could not change the channel on this live life TV show!

On the way home I insisted in buying some flowers. My wife loved purple Orchids. Purple Orchids were what I bought. We all went directly to her room after we had arrived. I gave her a kiss on the cheek and carefully placed the flower in the window sill. I wanted this flower to get whatever sun it could in the window and not wilt like our marriage. I was surprised to see that she did not resist the kiss on the cheek as she had done many times before.

What did that mean?

A few days later she told me that we needed to talk. This usually meant her getting a divorce this time. She would start a monolog about how stupid I was and that our kids are old enough to have their own lives. Then she would move on to saying all the paperwork is done and all I need to do is to sign and we will be done. She usually would end with "Life is too short. I have wasted twenty-two years of the best time of my life with you. Now, I want out. I had enough."

I was worried sick about the end of the world scenario, when she showed up to have lunch with me. I was thinking this must be serious. Maybe she really decided to end my miserable life. Maybe she is having an affair. But who in his right mind would want to have an affair of any kind with an iceberg?"

My wife Dian was serious and I knew she must have some pretty serious things to say. For God's sake she must have serious things to say since she had a notebook. It was even worse; she had her best friend "Deputy Rhonda" in tow. I was wondering if Rhonda was there as a witness for the delivery of divorce papers, or just as an assistant. I did not like Rhonda and I knew that this disdain was mutual. Rhonda had damaged and poisoned our marriage constantly. I knew her first husband. He was a decent man. Rhonda divorced him to marry her second husband. The second husband, however, happened to be a Xerox copy of the first and he had to go. Rhonda, being a paralegal knew all rights and legal angles and I knew that she was advising my wife all the time.

After some small talk, Rhonda started to talk first. My wife had shoved her notebook in front of Deputy Rhonda and she had just started to read a statement. I felt important. I looked like I was being interrogated for some matter of huge international interest that even network news was interested. But before Deputy Rhonda could put on her reading glasses, she started by saying that she knows that I do not like her. Immediately after that, she started to follow her notes. She did not really have to follow, but they were used as guidelines.

"We are here to talk to you about a serious matter. Your son Daniel is in serious danger. You as the father are legally obliged to do your best effort in helping your wife Dian in this grave matter." Hearing the Rhonda trademark words such as legal and best effort, I knew that as usual it must be Rhonda instigating this. Then I started to realize this was about my son. My son Daniel who was a high school champion in the sports; My son Daniel who just like Tiger Woods had always been a good boy; My son Daniel whom I taught golf to and who was my helper with car repairs and men things that we did together like fishing and going to Oshkosh Air Show each year for many years.

Shocked and surprised, I asked "My Daniel?" My wife jumped in angrily. "No dummy, it is our Daniel!" "OK, tell me! I am shocked! Daniel has always been a good boy. What are you talking about?"

It was Rhonda's turn to jump in this time. She told Dian to keep quiet. Then she re-emphasized, "Yes it is Daniel and it is serious!" My heart was racing and my entire life was being shown in front of my eyes as if another heart attack was imminent. Daniel and Debra were the apples of my eye. I loved them more than life. How could this happen?

Rhonda started to say something, and then Dian told her to "Shut up!" I was getting worried and angry. Dian started again. "Look, we have not been good example of married couples for these kids. Let us face it we have nothing in common and we should have never been married in the first place." After closing the book shut, she said what she really wanted to say.

She said "Daniel, your good boy, has made Lori pregnant. Lori is not pretty, and she does not even know how to be a mom. She is zero! She does not even fit your stupid five classes of women categorization. She is dumb, crazy, and on top of that she is out there to ruin Daniel's life." Then as if this was not enough, she added that "Daniel has dropped out of college!"

Rhonda, who had been painfully quiet all this time started to shake her head in disagreement. "Look Bryce, you had this coming. But it is not all your fault. Dian has to share some of it too."

Like a child asking for permission and advice, I asked "What should I do?" Dian did not wait even a minute. She raised her voice saying "Talk to your son dummy, talk to your son!" As if that was not enough, she said "Talk if you know how. I am not even sure you can do that. You never did that in our marriage!"

Pretending that I did not know any of this, I asked Daniel to meet me for lunch. He quickly finished his deep dish pizza and then said, "Dad, I have something to tell you. I am deeply in love! I want you to meet her soon."

I met Lori the next day at the same restaurant and again eating the same Chicago tradition deep dish pizza! She was intelligent, relatively beautiful, and clearly in love with Daniel. Daniel had an old and somewhat soiled shirt since he had started to work as a mechanic on a part time basis. However, Lori was going to college to become a journalist.

I asked what was most important for me first. "Daniel, did you drop out of college?" He was startled. "Come again. Dropped out of college, me? Dad this is my last year. How could I drop out of college?" I knew Daniel good enough to know that he would not lie to me.

However, I did not dare to ask the question regarding pregnancy.

A week later, I had lunch with Daniel again. Again, we had deep dish pizza the Chicago tradition. Daniel leveled with me. "Lori is indeed pregnant. I cannot afford to go to college and support her and the baby at the same time. So, I am seriously thinking about dropping out of college."

"Daniel, do you want my advice?" I asked. Daniel in a defensive posture said "It depends!" We continued talking for several hours. I know that I had made some in roads when he told me that he wants me to go the garage that he is working in. I was there the next day right after work. I had no choice. Dian had made this clear. Either I cleaned this mess, or I could not go home.

Daniel was tired and in bad need of a hot shower. Lori was four months pregnant by then. Daniel seemed angry. "Dad, Lorie has left me!"

I was desponded. But I did not let it show. I asked why? "She figured out that I had dropped out of college!"

By now Dian was desperate to somehow fix this so called problem. "Daniel, do you really love Lori?" His immediate response was "Of course!" "Then I earned my stripes. If you really love her, then go and ask her for forgiveness. Also make sure that you take some flowers with you."

I got a call the next day early in the morning. "Dad, she has agreed to come back if and when I go back to school. Now, what do I do dad?"

Let me call you this afternoon. I told him that I have deposited enough money in his checking account so he can go back to school and finish up his degree.

Now, I had the monumental task of talking to Dian. I decided to do this indirectly. I managed to be where Rhonda usually went for lunch. Without much embarrassment, I was able to share a table with her in this crowded restaurant.

I thanked her for her support and advice to Dian. Then I told her about what I had done for Daniel and asked if this was enough to keep Dian happy.

With a humiliating and childish laugh she said, "Dian? Can Dian ever be happy? Did you ever see her happy?" Then she realized that I was uncomfortable. She quickly changed the subject to reduce the stress. She was trying to linger and kill the time until she could politely bail out. She seemed to find this "coincidence" just awkward as I was.

As soon as I had said, "Sorry to barge in on you like this…"
She decided to give me the benefit of doubt. After all she had
never given me the time of the day for anything ever before. I
think that she must have felt a bit sorry too.

"Look, Bryce, you are a decent man. You work hard and you
try even harder to be a good dad and a good husband. But it is
not working!" Then, she started playing with the fork as if
shoveling the last pieces of the apple pie crumbs. She then
lifted her head just enough to look me into the eye. She
mustered all her courage to tell me "Bryce, just make sure that
Daniel does not make the same mistake in marriage as you did
in yours and I did in my second marriage!"

Then as if she was hit with something so bad that she was
going to cry, she excused herself and left the table. I felt really
bad. I had ruined her lunch and I must have hurt her some
way. The truth was that I had hated her all these years, but
maybe I was wrong by just listening to Dian and never sitting
down with Rhonda!

I called Daniel's University registrar, with prior permission
from Daniel. Contrary to what Daniel had thought, his status
was not "Drop out". At least, it would not turn that way if he
pays his tuition that he owes and penalties. When the registrar
calculated the figure, I thought he was kidding. The total
amounted to less than what I had paid for the pair of Pierre
Cardin shirts that I had bought at Heathrow Tax Free. I asked
if I could put it on my credit card. "Sorry Sir, we only accept
personal checks from our students or cash". That meant I
needed to take a cab and go across town right away.

There was a big line, but it moved quickly. I made the
payment, and proudly got the official University stamp and
Daniel was re-instated. At that moment, it felt like I had
conquered the world.

On the cab ride back and as I was rejoicing about my "generous" heroics for my only son, the cell phone rang. "Daniel, we made it, you are back in again!" Daniel was not happy or impressed. I could read in his voice that he was disappointed. He said "Dad I have a big test tomorrow. Thanks for doing what you did. I will pay back with interest. But it might be that I will flunk out instead of drop out! Sorry dad, I need to go. Got to go! Bye!"

Daniel called me the next day right after the test. He seemed to be exhausted but elated. "Dad, I think that I will not only pass, but might get a decent grade too!" Then as an afterthought "Dad you know that I am broke. So, this decent grade will cost you. You should have never saved me from dropping out of the college thing, now you have to pay…$65."

I have known for many years that God has a sense of humor. A $65 payment to a tutor that had coached him for the exam, the life saving exam at that, is what I normally pay for a decent business lunch. A decent lunch which does not include drinks! For the first time, I felt like the best dad in the world just because I had made Daniel happy.

A few days later I went Daniel's work place where he repaired cars. His boss, somewhat surprised to see me in my luxury car and expensive suite told me "Sorry I cannot shake hands with you. I do not want to make your hands dirty with brake fluid! But let me tell you this, Daniel is a great mechanic after having worked in my garage four summers! Customers like him and know that he always does a good job. In one case he lent his own car to a customer so he can go to a job interview while he repaired his car. He is a good man."

I waited for Daniel to wash up and we went to the nearest McDonald, where he usually went to have dinner with Lorie. Lorie's face seemed glowing! She sported a nice smile, and seemed to be pleased to have dinner with us.

"Dad, did you finish your book yet?" I had to be honest and say "No, I have had to put it aside for some time!" Then speaking with confidence the way he usually spoke, he added "Dad, can you believe it I have found my Roya and we plan to get married as soon as we get the old fashioned blessings from both sets of parents."

After dinner and some more talks, I extended my hand for a hand shake with Lorie. Instead she gave me a father-daughter hug! I was flying in cloud nine. I never had thought that I will ever see my grandchildren. Now I had a chance.

Daniel and his mother, Dian, had had a serious argument and by the time I arrived, I could see the anger and disappointment in Dian.

I convinced Dian that she should let Daniel and I go for a walk. However, she had had to have the last word. "Go for a walk and never come back, the both of you!"

As I was backing out of the garage, Daniel decided to open up completely. "Dad, I had found my Roya, and I wanted to marry her. I wanted to do what you did not get to do. More importantly, I wanted to have a marriage better than your and Mom! What am I to do? We took all precautions when we had sex. We acted as adults. Unfortunately we are part of that little percentage that is warned about pregnancy in spite protection!" I felt really sorry for my boy and now Lorie.

All of a sudden I realized that I have never told anyone about Roya. "Daniel, how did you find out about Roya?" Then just to drive the point home, "I expect you to keep it confidential!" He burst with objection "Confidential my foot, dad!" Then in a rapid-fire fashion "Roya is in your book. Not only she is in your book, she is in the first few chapters!" Then with puzzled and disappointed look in his face, he asked "Dad. Why did you chicken out?

"I feel betrayed. I never gave you the permission to read my book! You should have not read it! I could see that he was getting angry the same way an innocent man would look in a court being accused of something that he had not done. Almost yelling at me, he said "Dad you gave the book to me to proof read. Do you remember that? Remember all those crossing out and correcting of your grammar and spelling?" He was right. I was guilty as charged.

"I am really sorry, my man!" I told Daniel. Then it was my turn to ask a long awaited question. I asked "Daniel, are you sure this is your Roya!" Then to make it more precise, "Dan are you sure that you will not repeat my mistake?"

With a tone that could not be anything else except ridicule, he answered my question with another question. He asked, "Which mistake do you mean?" He was trying to clarify things "The mistake of not marrying your Roya, or the mistake of marrying my Mom?" Then with a sad voice, he said "Dad my mom is crazy and you are crazy too! Why do you put up with her?"

I started to answer both his questions, but I could not. What do I tell him? Then I thought of something daring and dangerous. I called Rhonda. Then, I explained the situation that we need as a matter of respect to get her blessings before Daniel, who is really in love with Lorie, to do the honorable thing and marry her. Unfortunately, Dian was dead set against this. Dian was dead set against and I could not wait to see my grandson or granddaughter before I died. I could hear Rhonda cursing. With some hesitation, she ordered me to let this part to her. She was going to have a talk with "That woman".

I parked my late model brand new car that I had just bought a few weeks ago, right next to Daniel's old beat up car. We had decided that we will go to Lorie's parents' house with his car. We did not want to show off our relatively high wealth to them.

This was a totally unexpected visit since Lorie was not there and Lorie's mom was in the garden gardening on her hands and knees. It seemed like Daniel had forgotten to call!

She washed up and we sat down for some coffee and cake. Their house was tiny compared to ours. On the other hand, there were flowers everywhere. Her dad was a retired paperback writer with a modest retirement that would be augmented each month with the book sales revenue. The house was spotless and books and bookshelves made it look more like a library than a house. Her father and mother were both well educated but their income was low. Her father had served in the Peace Corps in Chile for several years when he was young.

His father offered to show me the garden and his part that has yellow roses from Texas. Once in the yard, and quietly, he said "Congratulations for raising such a son. I admire and respect him. He is a good man and he will be a good son-in-law for me!"

When we came back I knew that her mother had given Daniel her blessings too. They both were enjoying a second cup of coffee. Daniel also had a sliver of second serving of cake so he will not ruin is fine figure. Lorie's mother was already mothering him.

Daniel had one more question to ask. He was asking "Dad what should I do?" After carefully considering alternatives in his mind, he asked, "Dad what would you do if you were in my place?" With as much assurance that I could give I told him "Daniel, you are doing the right and honorable thing! I would have done the same thing!" Daniel responded with "This coming from you, with your present marriage and your past with Roya, I do not know if this is a complement or an insult!" I decided to ignore this. He could be as sarcastic as he could so long as I got my grandson, or granddaughter. Rhonda called back to tell us that Dian has agreed to be civil about this marriage and she wants to know where and when.

A very simple wedding ceremony was arranged in a church near where Daniel and Lorie were going to live. Wedding dresses were made by Rhonda and they looked really nice. Apple pies for desert were prepared by Dian and Debra. And, of course, flowers were from Lorie's mom and dad including his beloved yellow roses of Texas.

A few weeks before the wedding, I got a totally unexpected call from Rhonda. After some small talk, she asked if we can meet for coffee. I did not want to do it, but I felt a huge debt of gratitude and an obligation. Furthermore, I was worried that Dian might have changed her mind about the wedding.

Rhonda started to say "You know that you owe me a great deal. I took Dain to a Doctor and she is now on Zoloft. You should see her less angry all the time. But this is not why I asked to meet with you."

Then she pushed back on her seat and said "As I get older my standards seem to deteriorate. I have decided to go back to my first husband. He always had a high opinion of you and you were partners at some point. Can you help me? Just ask him if he wants to have coffee with me. I am not asking for a date. I just want to have a cup of coffee with him. Is this a crime?"

They have been dating or "coffeeing" for several months now after I arranged that first blind date, or coffee. By helping make this wedding conceal the out of wedlock child, I think that I too am part of the American hypocrisy.

Six months and eleven days later, we had a granddaughter called, Dian Jr.! She was a seven pound feisty, noisy little bundle of joy with a temper just like her namesake.

From the minute that Dian Jr. was born, Dian was totally transformed. "Grandma Dian" was right in there to hold the baby after her mother and father were done holding and loving him. We spent a great deal of time in that hospital room.

It seemed like Dian was determined to give this slight barely more than five pounds premature baby in Intensive Care Unit all the love that Dian knew she will not get from Daniel or Lorie. I never forget the expression in Dian's face when she first laid eyes on this sickly little thing. Dian was alarmed, angry, disoriented, and discouraged, and stunned. After all this was the only one granddaughter that she knew she will ever have.

Dian Jr. being kicking and crying spunky dying baby had reminded Dain of her own self. This was a scene that broke my heart. Why is there so little love in this world? Why Dian did not get enough love and attention when she was a kid?

In less than a year, we were there again in what looked like exactly the same room. Surprising enough this time, Lorie was going through a C-Section after a high risk pregnancy with triplets. They were all boys, and one was considerably less healthy that the other two. Isaac, Tobias, and Abraham were my three new grandsons. Unfortunately, Isaac who was named after my father had a birth defect. He too had a heart problem just like my father and I before him.

After the birth of the three boys, Dian Jr. and Grandma Dian got even closer. Dian Jr. will spend Sunday nights with us. Then Grandma Dian will drive her to her kindergarten. Each week Dian Jr. will stay with us for three nights.

Dian Jr. even had her two rooms in our house as opposed to half a room that she had to share with Tobias in her house. One of the rooms had Grandma Dian's sizeable doll collection, and the other was re-decorated to be a typical bedroom for Dian Jr.

Grandma Dian and Dian Jr. had a great deal of fun together. I am positive that this was the primary reason for my wife's drastic change in becoming caring, patient, and most importantly mellow.

Dian Jr., also had another side. She did miss her mom and dad and brothers. But she did not miss all that bickering, fighting and shouting that was almost always present in their house. Dian Jr. was longing for peace and quiet. She was smart enough to know the value of harmony and togetherness. The other side of Dian Jr. would manifest itself in her sitting motionless and being totally absorbed in watching something. A sad feeling would then cover her innocent face and permeate to her entire being. Kids are smart. She knew that her mom and dad were not happy together. But I knew better. I knew that they had never learned how to be happy together and in a relationship.

The intriguing fact remained that Dian Jr. had complete power over Grandma Dian, although they were very close to each other. My wife, maintaining that Lori was not a good mother, had felt very sorry for Dian Jr. In addition our special needs grandson Isaac had also captured and ruptured Dian's heavy heart!

In one of our daily arguments, Dian had declared that she even had positive proof against Lori. "Look Bryce, Listen and listen well to what I am telling you! This woman Lori is not a suitable mother. She just has no idea what being a mother is all about!" Then she would go into an animated yelling. "She first got pregnant before she was married. Then she must have not been careful with her fertilization medication and that is why she had triplets. She is just no good. She is trying to destroy my Daniel. My Daniel is not the same Daniel that he was before he got married! I wish he had never married her! What the hell am I going to do with this Isaac? He looks retarded in addition to being sickly to me! I still love and adore him. What on earth am I to do?"

As years went by, Dian Sr. seemed to be more accepting of Loris and had less of rage towards me. Also, the tantrum and shouting episodes seem to be less frequent than before.

On the nights when Dian Jr. would stay in our house, we had developed a tradition. I would buy dinner from a different international restaurant, and we pretend that we are in that country. Japan, Hong Kong, France, and many other countries were our weekly choice. Of course this is all thanks to an infinite number of such restaurants in Chicago.

In the same room that we kept Grandma Dian's doll collection, which had become unquestionably personal property of Dian Jr. after she had adopted us, we had a big box full of international decorations. Yes, you read it right. Dian Jr. had adopted us as if we were her parents. There were so much unhappiness and fighting at home that Dian Jr. could not wait to come and stay in the relative peaceful shelter of our house. She would have her tiny suitcase ready and full of her things hours before we were going to pick her up. She would put her suitcase right next to the door and she would run out of the house just as soon as we rang the bell. Sadly, she would usually not be ready when it was time for her parents to pick her up. She would ask them to wait a few more minutes just so she can finish watching some program on TV, or to pack her bag, or to get a glass of milk to drink. Then she would quietly sit in the car for the entire trip back to her parents' home. In contrast, she would always be laughing and telling us stories or would be singing with us on the way to our house.

I remember that she had told her new kindergarten teacher that her parents were grandma and grandpa. The teachers had no problem understanding this since there were so many children of broken homes who lived with their grandparents. In addition they had seen us pick up Dain Jr. from the school a lot more than they had seen Daniel and Lorie. So, at least the new teacher was convinced that Dian and I were her real parents since we always gave her a big hug and kisses as we went to pick her up.

It breaks my heart when I think of this. A child should have a happy childhood with her parents. A child deserves a happy home. As heart breaking as this is, I forced myself to accept and understand this. I think that I would have done the same myself.

One hot and muggy summer when it was just too humid and hot for the elderly, infants, and people with a health condition to go outside, I met Joe. Joe pronounced his full Hungarian name so fast that I did not have a ghost of a chance to follow. As if having pity on me, he said, "I know, I know, nobody gets my real name so I go with Joe as my Americanized name!"

Joe was a thin man in a typical wool Chicago jacket that was better for a winter day. He had a nice shirt and a tie that was carefully knotted in a perfect European knot. By the way, it is easy to tell these two different types of knots. American style is more of a perfect triangle where all sides are more or less the same. The European knots are longer on the two side edges, and shorter on the bottom side.

His green eyes were covered by thick lenses of his professor like eyeglasses. Soon I was at a loss as to what to say. So, I asked him are you a professor? The response was somewhat baffling. With some huge regret, he said that "I was a history professor in Budapest. I wrote several books and published articles. Then, my wife insisted that we have to immigrate to the US. We did, and we had six happy years before she passed away and left me alone with nobody here."

Then with a fatherly sparkle in his eyes, he said, "Let me guess, you must be a businessman and very good at that. You must be very successful." I really appreciated his compliment. I had had a bad verbal argument with Dian that day and I had driven aimlessly until, I saw the library. Dian had gone into a rage threatening that she will destroy me. She had never said that before. A tirade of other threats followed the next fifteen minutes and I gently excused myself and left the house.

Joe was really interested in continuing the discussion that we had started. Something in his face said that he needed something, but he was too shy to ask. As any half way decent business person with interpersonal skill knows, sometimes people need some time to communicate the real issues. From his appearances, I did not think that he needed money.

Soon, he discovered that it was just better to tell me what he had in mind. "I am sorry to tell you this. I am one of those with poor health conditions. I should have never come out of my tiny studio apartment today. But, I did because it was scorching hot there today. My so called studio has only one window and there is not enough cross ventilation. It also gets about ten degrees hotter than outside. I came here to enjoy the free air-conditioning. The cab fare was a lot more than I had anticipated. So I cannot take a cab and it takes two buses from here to my apartment. Is there any chance that you can do I a favor and give me a ride?" Without any hesitation I gladly obliged since I had no place to go either. Usually I gave Dian about three hours to cool down before I dared to go back to home combat zone. I had another two and a half hour to kill. Since I was starving, I asked him if we can stop somewhere for dinner. His hesitations lead me to realize that he must be short of cash. "It will be my treat." This offer had not quite come out of my mouth before he agreed.

Just out of curiosity I asked him if he knew a good Hungarian restaurant nearby. He was only too excited to say yes. Then as if he had come back to life he added, "There is a nice one a few blocks from here that my beloved Lily used to love to go to. Unfortunately the prices are a bit high. But the food is excellent. The owners are Jewish and the place is clean and the food is out of this world."

When the Jewish owner saw Joe, he was elated. He greeted Joe as if Joe was one of Hungarian dignitaries. We were treated to an excellent Goulash and six other courses of a fantastic dinner. Dessert was tiny Debouche pastries. These pastries are made of rich ingredients and are just like nothing else in this world. There was also plenty of famous Hungarian Bull's Blood red wine.

During the course of dinner, Joe had done the best he could to eat slowly. But I could see behind that façade that he must have been starving worse than I was. When the main dish was being served, poor Joe did not know whether to inhale, or somehow consume the entire dish in just one byte.

The check arrived. The owner had given his VIP repeat customer a hefty 15% discount. Joe, offered to pay his share, and I had to remind him that he had agreed to this being my treat.

He had actually taken his valet out to pay. Without any intention to gaze into his valet, I was alarmed to see that he had one or at most two single dollar bills as his entire worldly possession that night.

I really felt his pain.

We had to jack up the air-conditioner to its maximum capacity to cope with hot and humid August day.

Joe was a lot more talkative now. He was jovial and I found that this frail man also had a sense of humor. Being hurt by my broken marriage, I asked him what made his marriage so happy. He proudly said, "My marriage was and was not happy. I loved Lily more than my own life. But, I did not like everything that Lily did. She had a brother who constantly borrowed money from me and never paid anything back. Also, Lily was bipolar. Only sad thing was that those days, we did not really know what being bipolar meant. Worse yet we did not have treatments that we have now. One minute she would be the happiest person and next minute for no reason at all, she would be the depressed and angry."

Then some million dollar advice came out. "Bryce, marriage like life is a gamble. Each day, it is a new gamble. Each day you roll the dice. Nothing can be taken for granted. Nothing can be promised. Nothing can be expected. Nothing is forever, expect for unconditional love. There is nothing to be had and there is nothing to be hanged on to." Then taking his time to carefully watch the traffic light turn green, he added, "All marriages are the same. They have ups and downs!" I was about to object and say, "But mine is always down. She is always angry. She always makes me angry and frustrated too."

I decided against venting off to him like that in our first meeting. Our father and son like relationship persisted for as long as he was alive. Just like Dian Jr., I too had adopted him as an assistant father. Or, Joe could be just a father who was a professor. I still loved and liked my own father. My dad was my dad. But there was nothing wrong with having a mentor father figure as well.

So, I could clearly see what Dian Jr. had done. She had adopted us with love. She had so much love that her biological parents were incapable of absorbing. We accepted her love, every bit of it, and appreciated it immensely.

One day Dain Jr. asked me if she was an unwanted child. I ignored this question pretending that I was listening to music. "Grandpa, please, please do tell me if I am unwanted." With all the courage I could muster I told her that she was not. I then bravely added that without her our lives would have been empty. I cheered her with the idea that she was our eldest granddaughter and that her folks loved her a great deal too.

Being extremely happy to hear this assurance, she nodded her tiny head. Then in an understanding way she told me, "Grandpa, I love you and grandma a lot too. Also, I understand why you love me more than others. You love me more because the others are boys and we all know that all boys stink. Boys are bad; they kick each other; they are spoiled just because they are younger!"

In our "International Box" in Dain Jr. room we had a lot of decorative items from Japan since I had travelled there more than ten times. Our favorite was a soup bowl with Japan Airlines written on it in shiny gold ink.

On the night that it was designated as Japan night, I had left work earlier to go to this excellent Japanese restaurant and get an impressive dinner. As it was customary, we would also try to learn a few words from that country's language each night. I found a Japanese phrase book published by Berlitz. We had a lot of fun pretending that we were in Tokyo that night.

Dian Jr. was about seven years old then. She gave us a lot of joy every time that she stayed with us.

I excused myself earlier and went to bed since I had a long trip to Singapore the next day. A United Airlines would take me from Chicago to San Francisco. Then I had to run from one gate to another and board the San Francisco to Hong Kong flight. Then with a two hour layover in Hong Kong, I would board my final flight to Singapore. It usually was less complicated than this. But this time we did not have any choice since this was a critical trip that was arranged with less than twelve hours of advance notice. I love San Francisco and I always wanted to live there. Unfortunately it was too late now. We had all our roots in Chicago. However, I had fallen in love with Chicago anyway.

I fell asleep quickly. I was dreaming that I was in Sheri's Ranch. In this dream, Dian had also come along. I was thinking with myself that this will be good for my marriage. Maybe this will help us rekindle our sexual desire for each other. All my usual inhibitions that would bar me from doing this when awake were pushed aside in this dream.

It was a fantastic dream.

I dreamed that I was fully aroused and sleeping on the bed in Sheri's with Gabriella standing next to the bed. Gabriella was giving my wife a lesson on makeup, how to please men, and sex. I was extremely hot for Gabriella even though I was deeply in love with my wife. However as the makeup and sex lessons progressed, I found my wife sexier and sexier. This went to a point that I did not know whether I was more sexually attracted to my wife or Gabriella.

I had told Dian many times that a clean and nice makeup is what usually turns me on. Also, I like femininity and gentleness.

I need to digress from this for a moment.

Deputy Parole Sergeant Crime Fighter Intimidating Rhonda had called me a few weeks ago. "We need to talk!" was all she said. Without any further questions, or arguments, I met her in her designated coffee shop.

"Bryce, you have heard of three strikes and you are out in the crime fighting! You, my friend have two against you, and I thought about giving you a notice before the third one!"

"Man, you are in trouble. Remember that Dain, in good faith and best effort ..." My stomach started to turn. This is the legal training that I had wished Rhonda had never gotten talking. Furthermore, this was coming as a shock. I had thought that we had made peace. I had stopped hating her for several months now. I was beginning to go into rage!

"Please do not panic. Let me explain. Remember that sport club and sauna appointment that Dain got for you?" Then without giving me any chance to respond or defend myself, she added her next sentence. "Do you remember that poor Dian flew all the way to Denver and got a bridal room?" I was beginning to catch my breath and I was trying my best to keep calm. Then with big pride and some arrogance she added "I talked her into doing all those thinking that sex will help you and your loveless marriage." "But you, a typical male messed it all up. Please do not deject her on her third attempt as that will be the end of the world!"

Now let us go back to my dream. I saw Gabriella then bend and try to kiss me as I was flat on my back on the bed. I asked her to please put on just a bit more lipstick. She did. I love the taste of fresh lipstick in a kiss, then she laid down right next to me so I could feel her supple skin and vacillating shapely breasts.

My wife was standing right next to us and observing all of these just like a graduate student observes and learns from professors. I was a bit apprehensive at first. Then I realized that this was for the good of our marriage and I had my wife's full attention and blessing.

For a few seconds, my eyes were fixated to the roof. Then gently, Gabriella's beautiful face appeared. She gave me a seductive and flirtatious look and then she kissed me very gently. It was so gentle that I barely felt it. Then she proceeded, while instructing Dian, to give me a French kiss." A delightful sensual moment passed by, and it seemed like Dain was curiously asking how it felt.

It was a nice dream. I was particularly pleased because in this dream, my wife had finally decided to learn to satisfy me. Of course, I knew how to satisfy her. She had told me that some several million times and I had really mastered it.

Then in the dream, as if I was in an out of body experience, I could see myself on the bed, and I could see my wife and Gabriella as well. By then Gabriella was lying on top of me and kissing me to make sure I was hard enough to perform. As passionate kisses progressed, I realized that I could not tell my wife and Gabriella apart. They had turned into one and the same person. The kisses were still very erotic. However at this point, I was trying to figure out what is happening. I frankly could not tell if it was Kat, Gabriella, Angelina, or Dian. Most importantly, it did not matter. They all felt the same in satisfying my urge.

A light went on and I woke up.

I was lying on my back in my own bed. My wife was right next to me. There was no Gabriella in the room. Then my wife turned off the light and we proceeded to have a mutually satisfying sex for the first time in about two decades that we were married.

This time it was my turn to turn on the light on the nightstand. It was Dian OK. She seemed to be somewhat relaxed and a bit, just a bit happy.

I turned around and mumbled something like, "Thanks Dain, this was good, really good." Then I kissed her on the cheek.

I woke up still somewhat satisfied, but late. I rushed to the airport only to realize my flight was delayed. It was delayed due to "Weather activity in Chicago!" I should tattoo this on my forehead since I have heard it so much. However, I was lucky. The delay on this flight had then made it mandatory for me to fly first class on another flight instead of business class just to be in Singapore on time for that urgent meeting. My manager had actually pre-approved it. We had outsmarted cold and windy winters of Chicago land, the windy city.

I had just made it to the United Airlines Courtesy Salon in Hong Kong Airport when my phone rang. The dial as I had preprogrammed it displayed "Rhonda the B." The B had been preprogrammed some time ago when I really hated her guts. The B stood for Bitch which seemed to be somewhat inappropriate these days after we had made peace.

I decided to answer it against my best judgment. After all I had a full two hours to kill.

To my surprise, I heard, "Hello Lover boy!" I had to ask her to repeat as I had never ever heard any complements from Rhonda. With some embarrassment and some delight she repeated what she had said and then added, "I hear you had great romance that was so hot that it turned the bed and your wife on fire!"

She was right. It was hot.

Then Rhonda told me, or more precisely demanded from me, to make her "Coffee-mate" to propose marriage to her one more time. Coffee-mate was a variation on the roommate that my wife had called me all these years. They were one level above roommate. Since they would only go for coffee that had made them coffee mate. According to this bizarre terminology, then if they married and had no sex, then they will be roommates. Roommates like Dain and I used to be.

However, one day Dian Jr. as an innocent seven year old had demanded to know from Dian why the grandma and grandpa that she had adopted as replacements for her mom and dad, did not kiss. She wanted an answer right there and then.

That was the same day that Dian decided to finally listen to Rhonda and do the night marathon.

As for Rhonda, she did marry again and as far I know they have happily become coffee-mates forever.

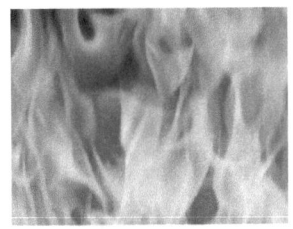

CHAPTER 25: Fire and Brimstone, Guilt, and Withdrawal

As I was inching closer and closer to what resembled normal intimacy for other couples with my wife, I hit a jolting road bump that nearly destroyed everything.

This road bump was the shocking reality that I had spent a lot of my money in addition to Pete's gift and I had been actually unemployed for several months. The unemployment tended to aggravate the severe "sexual addiction" that I had developed towards perfect sex in perfect settings and with the sexiest women in the world. Glamour, excitement, and the sex had intrigued and mesmerized and captivated me intensely.

The feeling was very similar to when I was trying to give up smoking. Right after a meal or at 10:00 AM smoking a cigarette was an unalienable right and highly deserved reward. I had to have those cigarettes at that time. Then when the phone ring, or as I was getting into my car, that smoking was another treat that I had given to myself for ages.

When I quit smoking cold turkey, I remember that just like alcoholics my hands would shake. I was experiencing the same emotional depravation earthquake. This was a tsunami that would shake my emotional stability from the foundation up.

Remember, before I had rationalized that those painted and perfectly sexy ladies that the media was telling me I had to had, were just not possible for me. I had made peace with not have much of sex in my marriage. Or, for that matter there was none outside my marriage either.

Therefore, as advertising media subliminally would drill in my mind that perfect sex is what I have to have and society said no you cannot have what everybody says you have to have I was caught in a painful depressing tug of war. Not having that ideal sex with that blonde on the motion picture screen, would really make me blue.

But now I had had that perfect sex with multiple blondes. Now the problem was I was missing that pleasure. I was getting depressed and sick.

Finally, I decided to use my thinking, and not feeling, brain. First my religion background jumped in. Since I had had intense enjoyment, pleasure, and excitement then I had to repent. I had to repent or otherwise there would be fire and brimstone. I could not dismiss this. I had to face this music. I had to sleep in the bed that I had made for myself.

The urges were getting stronger and stronger. I was daydreaming about how I can save, or even borrow money to go to my next escape and immerse myself in sex.

Even when I would go solo and manual each day, it was not satisfying enough. I needed the real world class sexy ladies. I did not seem to be able to function otherwise.

Then, I started to read the literature about sexual addiction. Some excellent work done at Stanford University caught my attention. The book argued that if sexual addiction is viewed the same way as alcohol and drug addiction, then the treatment can also be similar. The treatment would be a day by day reprieve and going to meetings and having a sponsor. Slowly, I started to get interested in the book. It had a twelve step program very similar to any Alcoholic Anonymous.

I started to make an inventory, of what I had spent. I continued by writing the time that it had taken me. Then I observed the urge that had intensified immensely afterwards. The net result was that I was spending a lot more time looking at online pornography.

Pete who had had the similar experience became my best friend and helped a great deal.

Gradually, I was able to find some other people in the Internet with similar situation and we became excellent friends.

It took quite some time before, I was back to being the same person I was before this.

Then one day, it seemed that if I kept my friends that I had found who had the same problem and called them everyday things would be somewhat less dangerous.

Charley had become an extremely valuable program friend. He would call me once a day. Also, I had a deal with him to call him before I did something stupid as a reaction to my sexual lust. He kept a daily regimen of writing in his diary and meditation.

My writing became a tool that helped me a great deal. Meditation was also powerful. It seemed that each day I was taking a baby step towards recovery. Sometimes, I would fail, but it was OK too.

One night, I got a call at 1:30 AM. It was Dian Jr. "Grandpa, please, please come to our house right away!" She hung up before I could ask why.

Upon my arrival, I saw two police cars. Dana Jr. was sitting in the porch with her suitcase and a bag that had a musical keyboard in it.

The police explained that there had been an attack on the house. A man had broken windows and the windshield of the car outside. "Dad, I had brought a colleague's car home to repair while I had lent her my own car. Her husband, who had been suspecting an affair all the time, thought I was with his wife. He got mad and did all these things." Then he went on, "Dad...", but before he could say anything else I took Dana Jr. with her suitcase, keyboard, and took her home to live with us forever. Whatever was happening, affair or not, domestic strife or not, I just did not want Dana Jr. to see any of it. She was quiet and scared during much of the ride. Then she said, "Grandpa, if you take me in, I promise to be a famous concert pianist. I promise that I will live a clean life and make you happy and proud."

Daniel and Lori never said anything about this!

There was also a gift in this process. I started to experience non-sexual love and practice it towards sexy women who were off limit to me. The one that I am most proud about is a glamorous sexy woman who works in a few cubicles away from mine. She has serious problems with her career, and I am able to talk to her about those, while she has been able to put things in perspective for me regarding sex.

We talk just the same way I talk to my therapist about sex. It is all clean and about feelings. It is honest and confidential. It is also helpful to talk to a member of opposite sex about these things and see from their point of view.

My friend Charley was quite concerned as my friendship and non-sexual relationship was developing at work. But, he has agreed that it is a good thing. However, he always cautions me that sometimes it only takes a few seconds to destroy the trust that she has given me.

I have learned long ago, that women are better able to talk most confidential things, including sex among themselves. Unfortunately as men, we feel weird and awkward. For a man to talk about his feelings, it is really difficult. We are trained as kids to face pain as a "man" and with stiff upper lips.

On one occasion, I told Charley that I was dying to go back to Sheri's ranch and party with anyone there. I wanted that and I wanted that very bad.

Poor Charley did not know what to say. Nevertheless he confided in me. He told me that he had never been to the high class scenes that I have been to. His specialty is to go to different dances and charm ladies by dancing. Then, most of the time, they are charmed and excited enough that they would not resist going to bed on the second or third date.

"Bryce, once I bedded them down, then I had to find the next one! There usually was no second time in bed with the same woman! In fact, after sex, I could not wait to say goodbye and go my way!" I had similar feelings towards sex. Unfortunately I was never that good on the dance floor.

One day, I asked Charley point blank, "What do you do when the urge is killing you?" His answer was that "I use the twelve steps' tools for recovery. I call my sponsor. I help others. Then as if he was divulging the secret that there is nothing wrong with relieving myself solo and manual. This gives me 98% of physical sexual pleasure with a woman to relieve my tension, and is 100% safe and trouble free!"

"Bryce, there are consequences in whatever we do in life. Bryce, I never forget how difficult it was for me to make amends to a woman that I had had sex with and who I had dumped the next day!" Then he grudgingly added, "I had convinced her the night before that I was in love with her. Worse yet, I had convinced my own self that I was in love. But minutes after we both had climaxed in orgasm, I was confronted with my shameful lie to myself and her. I did not really love her. I had told her what it had taken to bed her down. This is the height of my hypocrisy! "

The next day I felt like a piece of dirt.

I felt sorry for her and I hated myself. Was I that dishonest to do this? The answer was a resounding yes!

Pete had told me repeatedly that while what I had done was totally legal and even ethical, at least in the eyes of Europeans, I had not hurt anyone per say. I was ambivalent about the part that says I did not hurt anyone. However, I could not argue that I was on the road to recovery.

The silver lining in my seven months of unemployment was Dian's behavior. Sure enough, she threatened divorce but somehow she seemed to understand that I was hurt by unemployment. I had lost my self confidence and she could feel it.

She started to work like crazy and got all the overtime that she could get. She saved money any way possible. When she saw that I was grateful for these things, she would object by saying, "Do not get too happy, I am doing this for myself! You hear me? I am doing this for myself and not you." This was an angry woman's way of telling me that she loved me. She did not like everything I did, but that she was there for the long haul.

This scene usually totally confused Daniel and Debra. Nevertheless, this was love Dian style. This was what Dian had seen all her life between her mom and dad, her dad being a practicing alcoholic.

One day, I could not take all these things anymore. I picked up the phone and called Pete. "Pete, I am sick and tired of being sick and tired of unemployment, my marriage, and consequences of the wild living that I did when I had only a few quarters to live!" Then with a deep desperation, "Pete, tell me what would you do?" This usually solicited a sorrowful answer from Pete. "I hear you! This must be difficult. Take it as one day at a time. If you cannot, then take it as an hour at a time!" Then just to make sure he has done the best he can, he would add "Everyone has difficulties in life. We can overcome by taking them one step at a time!"

Usually, after having said these, he would then open a new chapter. He would then ask "What are your options Bryce? We always have options and choices to make." He will tell this as if life was a multiple choice test.

When I complained about how unfeeling and harsh my wife had always been, he would try to calm me down by saying "Bryce, the best thing to tell your wife, your better half, your lover is to say, yes dear! Now, do not get me wrong. You do not have to do it, but just say yes dear. Better yet, tell them, you might just be right. After all, who knows what is right and what is wrong! What has saved my marriage is that I do not fuss or argue."

I was experiencing a viscous cycle. I was urging for more of that perfect sex with the sexiest women in the world. This would make me feel more and more lonely, unwanted and hurt. Then, to sooth that painful hurt, I would long for sex and intimacy even more than before. I wanted to go get some more all the time!"

The cold turkey experience of giving up perfect sex with glamorous sexy women, combined with degrading feeling of being unemployed is an awful combination.

Furthermore, this experience destroys self confidence and respect needed to go on living as a normal person.

Interestingly enough, time can heal these wounds like all other wounds. I just have to give it time.

There is a Buddhism thought that says, the physical act of sex will never ultimately satisfy the desire for sex. This is according to Kusala Bhikshu. He continues that you could have sex 1,000 times. You will then want the 1,001st time and more and more. You could be ninety years old…blind and crippled…you still want to have sex. You will never get rid of your sexual desire by having sex. The facts are that the more you have the more you want.

According to Professor Stephanie Paulsell in a lecture in Memorial Church at Harvard, "Sex makes us regard the world with reverence and love if we focus on the goodness of body and be attentive to goodness of creation."

Also, according to Lisa Katz, "Judaism regards sex as being similar to eating and drinking. Eating and drinking are natural and potentially beneficial bodily functions. If done improperly, eating and drinking can become hurtful and shameful. If done properly, eating and drinking can be satiating and joyful. If done according to God's commandments (with blessings, a festive meal on Purim, four cups of wine on Passover ...), the mundane acts of eating and drinking can even be elevated to holy acts."

Nevertheless these experiences and teachings had helped me find some sort of peace and serenity with the sexual desire that can indeed be a furnace of heated and burning emotions.

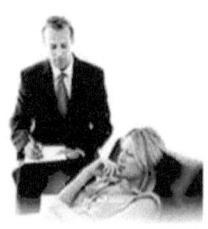

CHAPTER 26: Sexual Healing, Sex Therapy, Sexual Freedom, Serenity, Acceptance, and One More Thing

WOW!

This has been a wild ride beyond all my imagination! An old man defiantly relived his young days; an old man re-experimented with sex substance; an old man retraced past and found totally unexpected ending.

That old man is me!

While it was true that sex could have been equal to death as professionals had told me, I lived to tell about it.

I picked up the phone and called my good friend Pete. Without his generous gift I would have never gone on this escapade. His first question was, "Bryce, you are not dead. Are you?" Then right after that, "You did not go to Chapel of Love and get married while you were under the influence of heavy and perfect sex in Las Vegas? Please tell me that you did not!"

"The answer is no to both of your questions!" I assured him. After a long pause, he said that after I had left on my journey he had wished that he would have gone too. He would have wanted to go for the sake of good old days.

After I hung up, I went into deep thought, remorse, and some sort of delight all at the same time. As much as Pete had wanted to have gone, I started to question my own sanity for having pulled this stunt.

My Board of Mental Directors now jumped into high gear! "You should be ashamed of yourself, you dirty old man!" "Give me three, two, or even one good reason why you did this stupid thing! Are you crazy?"

That winter's first snow storm combined with heavy shifting winds made even walking difficult. My attempts to go for my daily walk, even with the heavy US Air Force Parka were "rendered impotent."

Darn it, I did not believe the self anger resulting from the combining the words render and potent together. "Damn it!" "Hell with render! I will erase it from my vocabulary forever. As I was trying to hopelessly find my way back in this relentless snow storm, with my lenses covered with steam, I realized that winter spelled out death. This is the same hellish death treat that had sent me on this tantalizing, yet gutsy trip. I found temporary solace in a store front that had a canopy. I was mourning the fact that I never made it to Mustang Ranch while it was open. I was thinking about that Ford Mustang from Roya that I never got. For that matter, I never saw my children that I was planning to have with Roya. Would these kids have had blue eyes? May be they would have had eyes mixing Roya's Blue and my greenish hazel color. Would they have turned out to be blond? Would I have been a happy father and husband?

How about the man in the Greyhound bus station in Reno? I was happy for him. He had retired and his wife and daughter were taking good and loving care of him. He was also very proud of the "Special Need" grandchild that they helped teach.

After all these years, I suddenly realized that my wedding ring was exactly the same shape and style as the one that the Greyhound bus station manager had that night that I stopped in Reno.

A wedding ring should have no beginning and no end. This is so, just like marriage. Marriage is supposed to have no beginning and no end. You get back to where you had started in a wedding ring!

It seemed to me that just like getting back to where I had started, I had re-arrived back at my youth. I had gone millions of miles on this mental, emotional, and nostalgic journey but I was back to where I had started from.

"What did I learn if anything? Is sex indeed overrated? Do men think about sex once every five minutes?"

A surge of questions along a heavy wind seemed to hit my face as I got out of the O'Hare airport to get into the waiting limo sent by the company.

Just like all those years in between that I had lived a dignified life and never did anything that was unethical let alone illegal, I had done the "Cash Register Honesty" rules and regulations in my life.

Even though my trip was a business trip from Chicago to London, I had carefully made sure that my four hour stop in Las Vegas did not add anything to the price of the ticket. This was my ethics and dignity working. I had done it right!

I had legal sex in a legal brothel. What is more is that I had respected the ladies and I had treated them gently and with kindness. As far as I was concerned they were workers. Workers just like any other workers. I was damned if I would judge them. They knew this when they saw it.

In fact, any of the ladies at Sheri's or other places can refuse to have sex with a particular person. They have a right to say no. This way they have their pride and dignity.

I remember a World War II movie that I had never forgotten. In this movie an American soldier who had not seen a woman in a very long time finds a sex worker. She takes him to her apartment. They set the fee, but before they can start he hears a faint voice. He jumps the same way he had done many times in the battle field, pulls his gun. All of these take place in a fraction of the second.

The woman keeps saying "No, No, No!"

The soldier opens the door and looks inside carefully. He was prepared to be shot at and he was equally ready to shoot. The woman continued saying "No, No, No! This is not what you think!"

The soldier sees a baby in a crib.

"Is this baby yours?" He asks gently from the woman. With fear tearing her apart, she says "Yes sir she is mine. She is only three weeks old and her father was killed four months ago!"

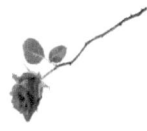 The soldier now has tears in his eyes. He feels relieved that there was nobody there to kill him as he had thought. However, he was asking God what a baby was doing in this hell of a war. A baby!

Without realizing what he was doing, he started to walk toward the crib. The mother started to plead with him even though had already returned the gun to its holster. "Sir, please, please, please do not go there." She said not knowing what he was planning to do.

The soldier brandished a big smile and suddenly returned to love and humanity after what had looked like a life-long absence, picked up the girl. He then gingerly cradled her in his hands. "I have one of mine too! Mine is a boy and he is in Boston. I have never seen him and already I miss him so bad I want to cry!" The motherly instinct by now had told her that she can trust this man. She cooked him a nice, but meager and simple homemade meal from her rations. He cherished every bit of the food.

As he was leaving the room, he asked if he can kiss the baby. The mother was glad to grant permission.

"Before I forget and go, let me give you this!" He opened an envelope full of local currency. This was the soldier's entire salary for the month. "You need this much more than I do." Then he pushed the envelope in her hands. She was refusing to take it, but he insisted.

Why was I remembering this now?

It seemed that I had done it right like that soldier. I had my own dignity and morality. I had never done something illegal. I had not done anything illegal even though I was deprived and longing for sex. I had done it right. I had done it my way. I was my own man! I had exercised "Cash Register Honesty!" I had never, ever hurt a woman to satisfy my sexual needs. Never!

"What?" "What are talking about?" thoughts poured in my mind.

While it was true that there were many illegal prostitution, there was still this hypocrisy that showed sex as the only important thing; showed graven images of the most perfect and sexy looking women; yet it also had laws that said you cannot have this! This was just like I had been sentenced to having only "quarters" to live; just like I had been told that sex is equal to death for me.

I seemed to suddenly see my dad in vivid colors.

I remembered talking to him when he was on his death bed. This was before I was even married. "I am not ready to go yet! I wanted to see my grand children!" He said with a few tears dropping from his eyes onto his boney cheeks. The ravages of his illness seemed to have eaten all the flesh from his normally jovial face.

"But dad, my engagement broke down two months ago. I am sorry dad! I wish I had given you and mom grandchildren. I am sorry. Dad, I, am really sorry."

I felt that, as the hero of the family, I as the miracle maker had failed my dad. This was my dad that I had loved so much. After saying these things, he started to go into this half sleep, half awake state that we had seen him do. My mom had made him his favorite dish. The French dish which is called beef Bourguignon. Then she had carefully put it into a blender and had put the semi fluid stuff in a clean plastic container. Under doctors' orders, my dad could only have soft food. In another tiny container, she had packed one of those tiny bottles of Burgundy that is served in airplanes. This was a souvenir I brought back from one of my numerous business trips to Paris. It also reminded us of our vacation to the Burgundy Provence in France one summer some thirty years before this. Once she arrived, she heated up the fresh grinded food in the stinky microwave available in the hospital. Then she used one of her most expensive plates instead of paper plates and created quite a presentation. A final touch of parsley and cilantro made the plate very presentable. The aroma and the site of the plate had woken up my dad completely. He quietly whispered to me "See all those French cooking classes finally paid off!"

My dad carefully ate every spoon of this food. Then, he motioned to my mom to get closer to him. "Thanks. I just wanted to say thanks. Remember, you used to make this food every Wednesday? I love this food!" Then with a voice showing love, remorse, and even depression, he added "I loved you before, and I love you forever. I ask all of you to forgive me if I failed to be what you expected of me to be." I had to leave the room. I could not take this anymore. Right next to my dad's room, there was a small court yard with a tiny garden and a worn out wobbly chair. I distinctly remember that I promised myself not to get to the end of life with having unfinished business. I noticed that my father's Doctor had found me. He had talked to all other members of the family except for me since I was on a business trip as always. I liked this Doctor. He was originally from Cuba and he had extremely refined manners. "You know that your dad does not have much time left. We have done everything we could do for him." Protesting what I had just heard, I asked if we could arrange for heart transplant. "Son, I am sorry to tell you this. That surgery will kill him! He is just too weak. He will not make it!"

My dad being an MD himself had sensed what I was feeling. He had read through my macho façade. He knew he did not have much time left. He knew that his death was eminent. He knew that he had a few days left. Astonishingly, he was at peace with this. He had accepted the fact that there is a time to live and there is a time to die. My dad was a hero since he had done many heroic things in his life. He also had heroes of his own. These were his mentors, teachers, spiritual leaders, and mostly intellectuals. He especially admired those existentialists who lived on the Left Bank in Paris. They focused their philosophical thoughts on the conditions of existence of the individual person and their emotions, actions, responsibilities, and thoughts. According to the Wikipedia on this subject, individual is solely responsible for giving their own life meaning and living that life passionately and sincerely in spite of many existential obstacles and distractions including despair, angst, absurdity, alienation and boredom. One day on a long bus ride from his office, he explained to me what he had learned from the existentialists, ala Dr. Condon style. He had learned that life is to be lived with maximum joy, passion, and mission for doing good. Then he would add, "Of course the million dollar question is exactly how? In my way, I have learned to just accept what I can accept and practice and remain consistent with my belief system. This is just for me. This is for me and no one else. This is just true right in this moment of time."

One of my dad's most admired heroes was an Air Force General. In fact he soon became my hero as well. We would visit this hero several times a year. He was a tall former US Air Force general who had retired by the time I was five or six. His face clearly showed a big scar from when he was shot down over occupied France during WWII. This very scar seemed to be more important to him than all the medals he had. This was a proof that he had the courage to fight the enemy. He had a nice house in Grosse Pointe, Michigan. He and most of his well to do relatives had always lived there. He was a few years older than my father and he loved all of us. The story is that some time before I was born, his oldest son Dwight gets very ill. Doctors tell him that his son was gravely ill. However, they told him that with some tough measures, they might be able to save his life. Their diagnosis was not confirmed by second opinion.

Story goes that my dad gets a call at 2:00 AM from his hero of all these years crying. After explaining the details, my dad tells him that he is on his way and hangs up. He had left his house in Chicago in such haste that he was not there to respond to all the following calls asking him not to go to Grosse Point.

My father appears in the hospital at 7:30 AM braving some awful winter snow storm. The story based on my father's heroic General goes like this. For a second opinion, my dad suggests a very famous Chicago Doctor. That Doctor's office tells my dad that they do not accept Insurance payments. They only charge cash. Neither my father nor the General had that kind of money right there and then.

My father excuses himself and goes to the nearest pond shop puts his wedding ring, gold watch, and a gold pen and pencil set on loan. Gets about half of what the Doctor wanted and calls and convinces the Doctor that he will pay the rest next day when he gets back to Chicago. The Doctor agrees to come.

It was not until 5:30 PM and pitch dark Chicago outside winter time that the Doctor arrives. My father had not left his best friend and his son even for a minute all the time. They had kept the son occupied telling stories of war, aviation and other things.

When the specialist arrived, he immediately recognized my dad as one of his colleagues who had read and suggested modifications to his latest paper. This being so, my dad enjoyed a great deal of kindness from this famous Doctor. Right about the time that the mother showed up from a long flight from Austin, a hoard of doctors and nurses and interns were standing outside the room to hear what the famous doctor had to say.

"This looks like what the first Doctors have diagnosed. Sorry about all that you must have gone through to bring me here, but this seems to be what they had told you it is. Unfortunately, there is no cure, especially if the fever elevates." Then he rushes out of the room discouraged and disappointed. About a minute later he comes back to the room and asks if he can make long distance calls from that room. The answer was no. Long distance calls could only be done from the pay phone in the hall way. Those days, you needed change. We all pitched in and came up with a huge number of coins to make the call possible. The Doctor swiftly disappeared from the room.

He re-appeared a few minutes later. It seemed like he could not make up his mind to either smile or be sad. His face showed both emotions. "Your son is gravely ill. But there is an experimental medication from New York that might, I emphasize, just might heal him and heal him quickly. Do you want to take the risk?"

The General stands up, looks out the window and comes back with "What will happen if we did not try this experimental medication?" The answer was "He will not make it, no matter what!"

"Then, what are you waiting for?"

TWA had a flight that left New York JFK airport with enough spare time for the medication to be carried in the special cooler. The flight took off and landed right on schedule with Captain Schiff at the controls of that Boeing 727.

The medication was administrated quickly. Then we waited for the miracle. The miracle, if it was supposed to happen, would happen quickly. The fever will disappear in about twelve hours and the patient will noticeably feel better.

The twelve hours came and went without any of the promised miracle. The General was "ordering" a second dose "Post Haste!" The chief medical Doctor told him that the second dose will be fatal. Either the first and only dose would work, or else there is nothing else they can do.

After about eighteen hours, there seemed to be a vague noise from the son. "I, I, want …" Then a second attempt he said, "I, and I, am thirsty."

He was on his way to recovery. In fact he had a full recovery. FDA approved that medicine about three years after this incident. My dad never had enough money to get his gold wedding ring, gold watch, or the gold pen and pencil set back and he never told a word of this to his General friend. My mother saved money and went to the same place and bought him a duplicate wedding ring with the words "LOVE FOR OO" engraved in the inside. The "OO" was to imitate the mathematical symbol for infinity.

My dad and the General became best friends forever.

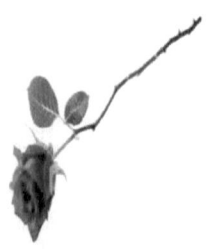

The General, being a handsome, daring, and tall man was married to an absolute "China Doll" and a "Nurse" classification who was a nurse during the war. She was a natural blonde with a poetic Southern Accent and a real delightful person to talk to. She too was tall and an excellent host. Their parties were just out of this world.

On my dad's last days, General arranged to go visit him in the nursing home. He had arrived before I did and I remember my dad's face was glowing with a big proud smile. "Bryce, General has been kind enough to drive all this long was to visit." Then looking at the General, he said "General, while I am so elated for your visit, you should have not bothered with such a long trip. I understand that you drove to Chicago." General quickly responded "But, Doctor you know that I love to drive." General had brought his son Dwight along. "Remember you saved Dwight's life?" Then quickly the subject moved to remembering the good old days of Baseball and the Wriggly Field and Chicago Cubs. General's grandson is a big fan. His name is Omar after Omar Bradley who was General Patten's Assistant. General has only one grandson, but this grandson looks and acts just like him.
General pointed out Dwight has never forgotten that my dad had saved his life. Then, there was a firm handshake. Before existing my dad's room, the General had a small flag of his World War II squadron that he had given to my dad.
As I walked to the parking lot with Dwight and General, he told me that had something that he wanted to give to me. He did know that my dad's days were numbered. He told me that my dad and he are both soldiers. He told me that he was proud of how brave my dad was in his last days. He then gave me a big American flag to cover my dad's coffin.

We used that flag, General's squadron flag, and several long stemmed roses to cover my dad's coffin. Among many guests who were there, the General, his wife, his son Dwight, and grandson Omar were all present. Before, they say goodbye to me, the General made sure that he told me that he lives by that Psalm twenty-three that was cited. Then with a voice full of grief, he said "Bryce, he might even be in a better place now. Please do not longer in grief. Your dad was a soldier and he wanted all of you to just remember the good times! Life is just too fragile and short!" When the General had passed away, we went to the elaborate funeral.

It seemed like half of Grosse Point was there. His son, with a strong resemblance to his dad read the eulogy. "My dad was a national hero. He fought in the Second World War and risked his life several times. On one occasion, his Flying Fortress was hit, and he landed heroically. He had a Purple Heart Medal and a picture with the president." Then trying to fight his tears, he added, that, he passed away with all his immediate family by his side."

Aside from all the heroics, his last words to us were "I love all of you. Remember, it is OK to be afraid. Then act as if you are not afraid. Live your life with as much courage that you can muster. I am not afraid of dying. I feel free. I did what was most important to me. I fought like hell in the war. I, also, fought like hell with this awful disease. Then, I even did that one more thing as well!" "That one more thing was to be my own man; live life my own way; bring beautiful children and grand children to this world and raise them to the best of my abilities. That one more thing was to be at peace with my life. Now it is time to say goodbye. I want to do this with courage and with peace." He died peacefully in his sleep.

I often think about that one more thing. Is it some kind of trophy? Is it some kind of accomplishment? Is it fame? Is it wealth?

The answer continues to be a mystery. What would my "one more thing" be? What one more thing would I think about on my death bed?

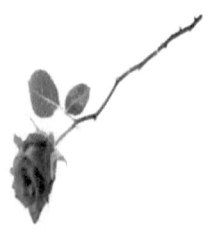

For my dad, that was clear. That one more thing was having grand children. For my mother that one more thing was to go back to her house for a few days and not die in a hospital room. This we tried but, she had become so weak that doctors strongly recommended against it. Instead she bargained with us. If I cannot leave, bring my older sister from Geneva. We did this one last thing. Her sister arrived completely washed up with jetlag and a long flight on Swissair. "Bryce, I am now ready to go home!" Mom, you cannot go home, Doctors do not allow it." She repeated, "Bryce, I want to go home, home," pointing to the sky with her tired and dehydrated eyes. Home! Home, where your dad is waiting, home! " That last home was the last thing we heard from her before she passed away with a gentle smile.

In her will she had written several times about her family and how much she loved all of us. In her will, there was a sentence that forbad grief and crying and encouraged us to celebrate her life. Just remember me in my best hour! Just think of the good times we spent in our most favorable vacation spot. Just remember all those episodes of 'I Love Lucy'. She loved to hear 'the man' play Babalu on his Cuban bongos. The man was Desi Arnaz, the real life husband of Lucy. My mother called Lucy's husband in life 'The Man' because he cheated on her. My mother and father had accidentally met in Omaha Orpheum Theater in the 40's in a concert by Desi. My mother loved Babalu that reminded her of the first time he saw my dad. We also watched all episodes of I love Lucy in Black and White and later on in color. We would change our lives around the "I Love Lucy" show time. I remember it clearly that after we had gotten our RCA Color TV almost all the neighborhood would join us to watch "I Love Lucy".

We had our weekly routine around "I Love Lucy". My dad would stop by at Andre Delicatessen on his way home. He would buy Salad Olive, Salad Legume, two freshly baked baguettes just like those you find in Paris and other things for our lavish diner while we enjoyed "I love Lucy". Usually, we would have one or more guests. It was fun. I miss those days. This was the last quarter of my life as sentenced by my doctors. They had said that "It is unusual that a patient survives more than the nine months."

Maybe the last quarter is up, but I am not done yet. I do not even know what my one last thing is.

I was feeling relatively OK for a man who had lived, and I mean really lived it up during the last three quarters of his live. "But, what now, what do I do when the last quarter expires?" I was repeatedly asking myself.

My "one more thing" was still illusive, conflicting, and confusing.

My children had grown up and they had lives of their own. Unfortunately at that time there were no grandchildren on mine. Nor, there was one to be expected within foreseeable future. My son was divorcing his wife for some reason or the other that I never really understood. My daughter and her husband had decided to be child free. Like me, they too have travelled all around the world together. The last I heard was, "Dad, why should I bring kids into this awful world? Just watch the news one evening. Dad, this world is so bad that I do not want children to see and live this."

My wife has made all the arrangements for my impending death. I could see that she loved me in her way and I could see that she would miss me after I was gone. However, she did not really want me to know any of these. She had a written plan for it all and she has hired my favorite catering company for food. They charge an arm and a leg for food and I won't be there to even get a taste. What a waste of money.

I will be buried in the same cemetery as my folks.

"Hell No, I Won't Go!"

My wife was cursing me. "You awful man. You were not much good in living, and you are not good even in dying!" I decided not to argue with her. She picked up the phone to call the Cardiologists number. I was wondering what she was going to tell them. Soon I guessed. She would tell them "This awful excuse of a man was supposed to have died by now, we have prepared everything including the catering, and he is not going!"

Fortunately, that was not what she told them. She asked for an appointment and promised to physically and personally bring me to the appointment, or she will kill me!" I figured I would be dead either way. So, there was no need to fight either way. She delivered me to the receptionist about thirty minutes early. Then, my wife left the waiting room crying.

"Bryce, how do you feel?" he asked. "Sir, I feel fine. No serious chest pain, no shortage of breath. No symptoms really and I painfully know that my last quarter is up!" He had a puzzled look on his face. "Aside from missing the last three appointments, I do not remember any quarters!" was his shocking reaction while still trying not to show his frustration. "Did you do the Angio?" he asked. "No Sir!" He stood back for a moment and looked at me as if I had disobeyed a military order and I had to be court marshaled.

This cardiologist is a Doctor's Doctor. He is a nice and caring man. He always wears ties that are from the best European design and quality. His office workers, assistants, and patients admire his ability to diagnose accurately and quickly. He was my dad's and Mom's Doctor. He had a book in his waiting room that was titled "Top Docs". This book was a few years old. Each page was a description of one of the best of the best. I had noticed that our cardiologist exhibited some of the behavior that was listed for the best of the best. His ambition for being the best of the best had increased my respect for him. I had utmost respect and trusted this man.

With dismay, he took his stat scope and listened to my heart. Then he hesitantly opened his notes. Right after that he ordered me to pull up my shirt again so he can listen to my heart again. I could easily see that something did not add up! I had always liked and admired this fantastic Stanford University educated doctor. He had excellent bedside manners. He asked me to promise to show up for a heart scan. No Angio, just a heart scan. No thread mill. All he wanted was just a scan.

Before he left the room, he showed me his notes. There was no diagnosis. There were "no damn quarters!"

I had two sleepless nights. Then it was time for the scan. It was painless and easy. We were directed to the waiting room, but we were told to stay there since the doctor wanted to talk to us after reviewing the scan results.

A slow and agonizing forty minutes lingered and finally it was time for the doctor to see us. This time they took us to a "Family Conference Room". The Doctor with a confident voice as if he had made another conquest over his nemesis, the internist, had an announcement to make.

"Bryce, I never told you about any quarters, and there is no notation here. This is the good news. However the bad news, and what I profoundly apologize for, is that another person's diagnosis was faxed to us by the internist. The names are very similar. Then he proceeded to show the first proof. "See, these are holes made by the staple. The first page which has the patient information is indeed yours. Now, look at the second page. Please look at the staple holes carefully. The first page the two holes were parallel to the top. In the next two pages that must have been sandwiched in with the other pages have staple holes that are almost vertical. Now, please look at the bottom. Your Patient Identification Number or PIN is BDC22894336. Of course BDC stands for Bryce Daniel Condon. Look at the two pages sandwiched in between. The PIN Number is BDC22811308. However the last page is truly yours." After some careful reorganizing the folder, he promised to clear this up. Then as if he was just equally hurt, he added "I might have made the same mistake. However, I would have definitely cleared this up had you had kept your appointment!"

He then shook my hand just as hard as he could. I could see that he was elated to have authoritatively and accurately have given diagnosis. For me this was a diagnosis that meant life rather than death.

The word sandwich generation had made me nauseated. I had always been upset as belonging to the so called sandwich generation. Then as if that was not enough, now the sandwich effect had turned my life upside down and topsy-turvy. My anger about the first sandwich syndrome is legitimate. However, my frustration about the medical document sandwich is a mixed blessing and a sort of curse at the same time. It was the most pleasurable time of my sex life. I feel younger, and alive. It also is a curse because I did things that the more conservative Bryce would never do.

For that matter who knows, maybe this sandwich mistake was what I needed to come back to life. All that fearless wild living might be a good lesson for me that fear is one of the worst four letter words in English language.

This whole mistake and the reckless, yet extremely pleasurable living was not that funny, amusing, interesting, or even something that I wanted to hear after all that wild living that I had had done.

My wife was furious. She had to cancel all those elaborate plans for my funeral.

Before, I left my Cardiologist's office; he asked me if there was something that I wanted to tell him? My honest answer was yes! In a few sentences I told him about my escapade. Then I summarized by saying that I was always protected. This means that I always used condoms. I know that as a physician he would be concerned about AIDS.

Being a world class doctor, and a top doc at that, he shared with me that he had done similar things. Then he added that his was with a motorcycle! His father being also a doctor had forbidden him to ride motorcycles since his uncle was killed in an awful motorcycle accident. Then as if he was making a confession, he added that after his own marriage broke up, he bought a top of the line motorcycle, found his high school sweetheart and the "Hot Riders, or Suicide Jockeys" as Ham Radio operators used to call them those days. I travelled the entire Highway 1 from Northern California to as far south as it went.

As he had realized that he had spent too much time about the nostalgic past, he got up and closed the door to his office. He seriously told me that "I have a suggestion and it is just a suggestion. Make sure that you get an AIDS test. Some condom tests have shown that AIDS virus can penetrate through a completely new condom. It does make some scientific sense. The diameter of AIDS virus is less than the molecules of the rubber compound used to make the condom." Then before he opened his office door, he said this is a man to man talk and it was beyond the scope of my regular heart treatment. Then as a second though he asked, "What was the name of the place in Las Vegas?" He wanted to know this just for the reference, especially since he has become single again.

This is now few years later, and several "routine" appointments later. I am still alive. I have even figured out what my "One More Thing" is.

I want to go in peace, in my own bed, with just my wife and children by my side. I have no idea when that day will be. However, I have realized that although I do not like everything about my wife, I love my family dearly. And for my brothers and sisters, I would like them to also join us, if they can.

Most importantly, I want to hold my son, my daughter and my wife's hand in my last minutes before I go home to join my beloved mom and dad. I want Babalu, Hot and Spicy, and It is a miracle from Jefferson Airplane, My Love from Petula Clark, and Edith Piaf's "I have no regrets" in its original French language to play on my iPod.

Babalu as it was the music that introduced my mom and dad together.

Hot and Spicy to describe those last quarters of my life that I did not give up joys of life. Indeed I lived up all my fantasies of having sex with the most beautiful women in Red Light District, and later on in Sheri's Ranch under most ideal conditions portrayed in the movies.

The only regret was that I realized how empty all of these can be.

"I have no regrets" depicts my life's lesson to be brave and not to fear. Life is a joy, and in spite all the movies and graven images in Hollywood, there are colors that are real and there are those that are not. I am proud that I was real and honest to myself. I, indeed have no regrets!

Jefferson Airplane's Grace Slick's song is right. Life is a miracle. Our entire being is a miracle. Love is a miracle.

Then, please play my first love in songs, Petula Clark's music. Petula Clark that I saw her sing "My love" in Olympia Theater in Paris and Petula Clark whom I flew to San Francisco in 2008 to see in her concert. I want to leave peacefully and with love. Love of my loved ones is very precious to me, even if things have not been perfect or even good all the time. I want to tell my wife, kids, grandchildren, brother, sister, and all those who had come in contact with me, friends, colleagues, everybody and everybody that I loved them and I loved them dearly.

Love can be one of the most powerful human joys even if there is sometimes pain. Also, when love is considered, even a 100 year old Forrest Lunsway was not too old to ask the 90 year old Rose Pollard to marry him. They had both lost their spouses, and they had dated for 28 years until, finally, Forrest asked his girlfriend that he was in love with to marry him! It took him 28 years after they first had met in 1983 to pop the question. While they were dating all those years, Rose had told Forrest that she had no intention of marrying again. A decade or so later, Forrest decided to have the courage to ask why they never had married each other? She responded, "Well, dear, you never asked!"

Right after that, he quickly got on his knees and popped the question.

She said yes! After the wedding Forrest told reporters that he plans to live to ripe age of 110 since he had just gotten married at the age 100.

I want to leave this world with all my four grand children near me and with love.

REFERENCES:

1. Out of the Shadows: Understanding Sexual Addiction - Paperback (May 23, 2001) by Patrick J. Carnes

2. Facing the Shadow by Patrick Carnes

3. Afternoon Delight: Erotica For Couples by Alison Tyler (Feb 10, 2009)

4. The Full Color Guide to Sexual Pleasures from A to Z - Paperback (1979) by Gunther Hunold

5. Intimate Kisses: The Poetry of Sexual Pleasure by Wendy Maltz and Thomas Moore (Dec 12, 2003)

6. In The Shadows of The Net: Breaking Free from Compulsive Online Sexual Behavior [Paperback].

7. Patrick Carnes Ph.D. (Author), David L. Delmonico Ph.D. (Author), Elizabeth Griffin M.A. (Author), Joseph M. Moriarity (Author)

8. Last Tango in Paris Starring Marlon Brando, Maria Schneider, Maria Michi, et al. (Nov 3, 1998)

9. Lie With Me (2005) Lauren Lee Smith (Actor), Eric Balfour (Actor), Clément Virgo (Director) | Rated: Unrated | Format: DVD

10. Guide des jolies femmes de Paris de Pierre-Louis Colin (Broché - 10 avril 2008)

11. The Graduate Starring Dustin Hoffman, Anne Bancroft, Katharine Ross, et al. (Apr 5, 2005)

12. Splendor in the Grass (2009) Natalie Wood (Actor), Warren Beatty (Actor), Elia Kazan (Director) | Rated: NR | Format: DVD

13. Irma La Douce Starring Jack Lemmon, Shirley MacLaine, Lou Jacobi and Bruce Yarnell (2001)

14. Avanti! (1964) Jack Lemmon (Actor), Juliet Mills (Actor), Billy Wilder (Director) | Rated: Unrated | Format: DVD

15. Days of Wine & Roses Starring Jack Lemmon, Lee Remick and Jack Klugman (2010)

16. Sexus (Sub) [VHS] Starring Willy Braque, Yves Duffaut, Annie Josse and Virginie Solenn (1999)

17. Some Like It Hot Starring Marilyn Monroe, Tony Curtis, Jack Lemmon and George Raft (2001)

18. Lonely Planet Amsterdam (City Guide) by Karla Zimmerman, Caroline Sieg and Ryan Ver Berkmoes (Paperback - Mar 1, 2010)

19. Madam: Inside a Nevada Brothel (Society Culture General) [Paperback]

20. Madam: Chronicles of a Nevada Cathouse [Hardcover], Lora Shaner

21. Plane Insanity: A Flight Attendant's Tales of Sex, Rage, and Queasiness at 30,000 Feet - Paperback (Feb. 5, 2003) by Elliott Hester Plane Insanity: A Flight Attendant's Tales of Sex, Rage, and Queasiness at 30,000 Feet - Paperback (Feb. 5, 2003) by Elliott Hester

22. The New Joy of Sex (The Joy of Sex Series) by Alex Comfort (Oct 1, 1992)

23. The Men's Health and Women's Health Big Book of Sex: Your Authoritative, Red-Hot Guide to the Sex of Your Dreams (and His!)/ Your Authoritative, Red-Hot Guide to the Sex of Your Dreams (and Hers!) by Editors of Women's Health and Men's Health Editors of (Feb 1, 2011)

24. Men's Health Guide to the Best Sex in the World by Men's Health Editors of (Nov 11, 2008)

25. Rekindling Desire: A Step by Step Program to Help Low-Sex and

No-Sex Marriages by Barry W. McCarthy and Emily J. McCarthy (Jan 15, 2003)

26. Testosterone for Life: Recharge Your Vitality, Sex Drive, Muscle Mass, and Overall Health by Abraham Morgentaler (Oct 27, 2008)

27. Schooling Sex: Libertine Literature and Erotic Education in Italy, France, and England 1534-1685 by James Turner (Mar 27, 2003)

28. Risky Lessons: Sex Education and Social Inequality (Rutgers Series in Childhood Studies) by Jessica Fields (Aug 30, 2008)

29. Brothel: Mustang Ranch and Its Women - Paperback (June 25, 2002) by Alexa Albert

30. The Forbidden Apple: A Century of Sex & Sin in New York City by Kat Long (Mar 1, 2009)

31. Sugar Blues [Mass Market Paperback] William Duffy (Author)

32. Arizona (2003) - Audio CD by Mark Lindsay

"I loved every moment of being with you even though we were together for such a short time. I am sorry about things not working between you and Roya and that wedding dress from Gallery La Fayette. I promise to make it up to you on our next time together!"

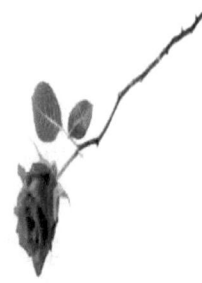

www.ingramcontent.com/pod-product-compliance
Lightning Source LLC
Chambersburg PA
CBHW061339280526
45784CB00001B/62